Peas, "Pills," and Parkinson's

ALICE CROOKER

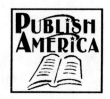

PublishAmerica
Baltimore

ISBN: 1-4241-3729-2
PUBLISHED BY PUBLISHAMERICA, LLLP
www.publishamerica.com
Baltimore

Printed in the United States of America

INTRODUCTION

You or someone you know has a problem. I am sorry! Since I cannot fix your unfortunate situation, I wrote this book to cheer you up.

All proceeds will be donated to The Virginia Mason Foundation to help improve the lives of Parkinson's disease patients.

I used to be a storyteller. After church one day a distinguished businessman approached me and said that if I would make tapes of my stories he would sell them for me. I am not very fond of the sound of my voice, so I decided to write a book instead.

It is amazing what a few words of encouragement can do for a person, and I undertook the writing of this book largely because of this man's encouraging words.

Unfortunately, he has been severely afflicted with prostate cancer. We all hope and pray that by the grace of God he can somehow win the battle with this disease.

I have Parkinson's disease and I know I could have adjusted to it much easier if it had simply waited to afflict me, say, about 10 years after I had passed away. I deeply admire and respect those who readily accept Parkinson's and actually say they are glad they have it.

I am not yet at that stage. I wonder if I ever will be.

You may have heard about Parkinson's from the celebrity's point of view. I would like to tell you what it is like for the ordinary, everyday obscure person – before and after the diagnosis.

I hope you will gain courage from my story and that it will help you deal with your particular "monster" in a positive manner.

Please don't think, "Oh help, here's another of those 'attitude' books where everything turns out for the best if a person just manages to laugh long enough." Unfortunately, it isn't always easy to laugh at Parkinson's. The feeling that some things in life just aren't fair keeps intruding.

I do not have many answers to the challenges of life, but I do believe with all my heart that with God, guts, good doctors and as much humor as we can muster we can all make it through anything.

No one, no matter what their circumstances, needs to give up. I can truly say that my extremity has been God's opportunity.

Did God hear and help me because I am special? Yes, because to Him we are all special. I am an ordinary person. I can be abrasive, and anyone who knows me will readily attest that I am far from perfect. Why then did God help me? The answer is simple: I asked Him for help!

ACKNOWLEDGEMENTS

First and foremost is my faithful, level-headed husband, Dave.

As I sat at his retirement party – a celebration of 36½ years of continuous employment with Plum Creek Timber Company, I saw how special he was, not just to me, but to all those in his workplace as well. I was thrilled to see that I was not alone in my admiration of this man.

Our children, Becky Alice DeOliveira and Daniel David Crooker, are a source of great pride to both of us and we are pleased with their excellent choices of spouses, Japhet and Stephanie who like us, visit us and travel with us.

It goes without saying that our grandchildren, Joshua and Jonah, are the finest, with their big chocolate-brown eyes and wonderfully happy smiles. They were a strong motivator to keep living.

My parents were the best for me. Life is much easier after watching them battle away for years to get a drop of water or to start their car. They could have had a life of leisure, but what would I have learned from that?

I wish the best for my troubled brother, Victor Shumate. May he recover sufficiently to enjoy a fine meal once in a while and stop worrying about all the people who are eating three squares a day. May the good Lord bless and keep you, Vic, wherever you are and whatever you are doing.

A special thanks to my amazing mother-in-law, Adaline Lane, who is still working in a nursing home at age 85. She took me to the doctors and brought me breakfast and good cheer.

My admiration goes to my patient father-in-law, Lawrence Crooker, who though hardly ever sick a day in his life, suffered a devastating stroke two weeks before his 80th birthday and has been disabled for nearly 10 long years. None of this was his fault or choice, yet he still smiles and never complains. His wonderful and faithful wife, Elsa, continues to work tirelessly so his surroundings are always immaculate. They have shown great interest and support for this book.

My gratitude to dear Auntie Mildred Smith, without whose Irish spunk nothing ever would have been accomplished in my family. She is the most amazing person I have ever met and is still energetic at 90.

My cousin, Gloria Sexton, is an angel. She called me faithfully and encouraged me mightily

My kind and understanding boss, Edward Basoglu, always reminded me that God would take care of me—he was so right!

Ken and Shirley Gregory, who, in spite of numerous personal tragedies and many health problems of their own, have never failed to be upbeat and helpful.

Our reliable friends George and Martha Hoffmeister who never forget us, or anyone else who needs a helping hand. Martha has uncommon, common sense and so does George. Furthermore, they are fun.

Jack and Nadeen Irvine helped me greatly by allowing me to help them. May God bless them and keep them.

Thank you to Jim and Sheryl Learned, our close friends of many years for having their entire church praying for me.

Pastor Phil Lizzi and his wife Judy made a special effort to arrive at the hospital in the wee hours to pray for me before my surgeries. Their caring and encouragement helped a lot.

Carol Minami kept me going with her quiet thoughtfulness— even left me a much appreciated green cozy hat for my bald head.

Don Murphy, CPA, wrote me such a kind, caring note, I still have it stowed away in a safe.

Wyn and Waltraud Pauly are unique, longtime friends. Waltraud and I have walked nearly 2000 miles together—we also solved every major world crisis to our satisfaction.

Dr Stanley Ray and his wife, Florence never failed to look me up when they were in town to bring me flowers and good cheer.

Vern and Twyla Schwisow never gave up on me—always came to see what was going on and generally kept track of us.

Virgle and Carolyn Seaton are wonderful friends who worked with us for years with the children at church. They moved to California several years ago, but their e-mail messages have provided encouragement and it is a bit of "heaven on earth" when we are fortunate to be with them.

Jizel Wanaka, is a hilarious friend and co-worker with enough spunk and humor to brighten any day no matter how dark.

Precious members of the Kirkland and Bellevue, Washington and Stanborough Park, England Seventh-day Adventist Churches who prayed for me—it worked.

I owe much to the many physicians who patiently diagnosed and expertly treated me:

Dr Eiji Minami, a quiet, careful excellent surgeon.

Dr. Peter Nora has a steady hand and kind heart.

Dr. Geoffrey Jiraneck is a man of action, who doesn't mess around. Once I saw him, my medical mysteries began to unravel, because he saw all of me, not just my troubled innards.

Dr. John Roberts, the king of all neurologists – where he goes, I will follow.

Dr. L. William Traverso a great surgeon with a great sense of humor. I felt a kinship with him.

Dr. Anne Tuttle, my patient and kind internal medicine doctor.

Roberta Kelly, the wonderful speech therapist at Virginia Mason Hospital.

Dr. Russell Vandenbelt, a true friend who saved my life by referring me to Dr. Jiranek.

Many thanks to University of Washington Medical Center ER Doctors, especially:

Dr. Frank; if I should ever have a heart attack, this is the man I want to have working on me.

Dr. Russell McMullen, a wonderful, kind, genius, who helped us through a difficult time.

Fellow DBS survivors and their caretakers: Wendy Fielding and her husband Lynn, Don Goodman and his wife Jan and Dick Skordal and his wife Virginia. Dave and I feel a strong kinship with these wonderful folks, because they have been "there."

A huge thank you belongs to MEDTRONICS CORPORATION for providing the science and technology of hope.

Blessings also to the fine medical staff of the Volunteer Fire Fighters at STATION 22 in Kirkland, Washington. They always came and tried to help, never told me I was crazy, even though I sometimes thought it must be so.

I am very grateful to Publish America for offering to publish and promote this book. I steeled myself for the rejections and sincerely hoped the battle to publish this book would be easier than the battle to live and write it. They pleasantly surprised me with a contract. They have been so patient and easy to work with and have made my dream come true.

I cannot adequately express my thankfulness to Don Duncan and his wife Mary. Don has spent hours, days and weeks editing this book. Don's credibility and expertise have added immeasurably to the success of this book and his encouragement kept me going. One would have to see the dedication of this wonderful, loving couple to believe it – a true Christian example to us all.

Last, but certainly not the least is Virginia Mason Hospital in Seattle, Washington. Yes, the doctors are wonderful, but they wouldn't be able to do much without the hospital facilities and incredible staff. Even their gift shop exceeds all expectations.

Contents

Chapter One

THE WARNING SIGNS

My dearly beloved husband Dave obviously was having a mid-life crisis! Why else would he suddenly start following me around, complaining about the way I walked?

I had been walking for years, and I certainly didn't need him to tell me how to put one foot in front of the other. What was the big deal about something as automatic as walking?

Looking back, I realize Dave was aware of a growing problem. But I was simply too busy or too stubborn to listen to him. In addition to working full time, I chaired our Church Board, did the housework and walked four miles four times a week.

With all that on my mind, Dave was concerned about something as inconsequential as my failure to swing my left arm when I walked. He had gone so far as to offer me "walking lessons." What foolishness!

Our two children had recently flown our warm and cozy nest to become college students, and Dave and I were trying to adjust. Becky and Dan had brought joy, laughter and assorted crises to our home for years. Now the only reminders of their existence were colossal tuition and housing bills.

Unlike the children of our friends, ours not only didn't live nearby, they didn't even live on the North American continent. Becky was attending college in England when she fell in love with and married Japhet De Oliveira. That prompted Dan, who was very fond of his sister, to decide he also wanted to attend college in England.

Becky's wedding in England had been straight out of a fairy tale. I sewed her wedding dress in my spare time and planned vacations for us and for Dave's parents, who accompanied us to the ceremony.

After the children left, Dave and I threw a huge "pity party" for ourselves. Dave took to snarling "Shut up!" at the neighbor's barking dog. I wallowed in misery, since all I had ever wanted in life was to have children.

My health, previously labeled "perfect," seemed to be going downhill fast. Even my teeth were a problem. Our dentist took an overly long look in my mouth and said, "It looks like you will need a root canal. You have an abscessed tooth. Take this antibiotic."

When I told my friend Cherry about the problem, she said, "Root canals are terrible. You will have an awful time."

I replied, "Give me a break. I've had back surgery, so this root canal will be nothing."

I was wrong. She was right. The root canal was worse than "terrible." It had to be done four times. That's right, four times! The final time, the dentist pulled the abscessed tooth and replaced it with a fixed bridge, which I – trying to maintain a sense of humor – decorated with a portrait of Mickey Mouse.

Call it a case of arrested development if you will, but my entire house is decorated in a Mickey Mouse theme. Walt Disney must be smiling down on me. I should note that as I tried to get out of the dentist's chair, after the third attempt at a root canal, the dentist said, in a worried tone,

"Are you going to go down?"

"I don't think so," I replied. "Have you ever had anyone fall over?"

"Not so far," he answered.

That comment and Dave's worry about the way I walked got me to wondering why I had become so unsteady. I wasn't exactly old, just 49. But in addition to a lack of arm swing and poor balance, I had also begun to notice a tremor in my left arm and left leg.

While Dave was on a business trip to Japan, I catalogued all my symptoms and the conclusion I reached petrified me. "Alice," I said to myself, "I'm afraid you have Parkinson's disease."

I immediately started reading up on Parkinson's, an unpredictable and incurable brain disorder. It is caused by the death of the *substantia nigra*, the area of the brain that controls movement. By the time symptoms appear about 80 percent of the *substantia nigra* has been destroyed. No one knows what causes the disease.

I told a nurse friend of my self-diagnosis and she said, "That's ridiculous, you are far too young for that." I was so pleased by her response that I told another friend I was so glad I didn't have Parkinson's that I didn't care what my problem might be.

That was my mindset on "Doomsday."

Chapter Two

DOOMSDAY

The charmed life I had taken for granted came to an abrupt end two days before Thanksgiving 1996. I still find it hard to describe the hurt and outrage I felt upon being formally introduced to Parkinson's disease or simply PD.

I was in the office of a physician specializing in neurological diseases. His office was in upscale Bellevue, Washington, the fast-growing city east of Seattle, across Lake Washington. At the end of an hour-long neurological examination, he pointed to a chair across from his desk and said, "Please sit down and we'll talk."

I took a seat and waited for him to say some of the things I was desperate to hear.

Such as, "What's eating you anyway? Can't you see that I'm a very busy man with many people to help? Why don't you get a hobby and enjoy yourself and be thankful you're such a fine specimen of health and vitality. Certainly you can find something better to do with your time than to sit around imagining you have a horrific health problem. You are a textbook hypochondriac! I've never met anyone as self-centered as you."

Instead, without mincing words, the doctor said, "You may continue to work and you will be 'all right' for about 10 years. You have Parkinson's disease."

If he had thrown a bucket of ice water on me, or poked thumbtacks straight into my eyeballs, he could not have done more to shatter the fantasies I had dreamed up to shield me from the dreaded diagnosis.

I burst into tears. Still grasping at straws, I said, "How do you know that I have this disease?"

His reply: "I knew it the moment you walked through the door!"

"Now isn't that just great!" I whined. "When I'm walking around people can just look at me and say, 'She has Parkinson's disease.' Why didn't anyone bother to tell me? I will furthermore inform you that I have been an active person and nearly climbed Mt. Rainier. I would prefer to have a brain tumor."

Did he apologize and say, "I had no idea you would be so offended. If you'll give me another chance perhaps I can come up with a diagnosis more pleasing and convenient for you." Of course he didn't. Instead, he handed me fistfuls of Kleenex. Then he asked if I'd been afraid I had Parkinson's.

I replied that I'd been petrified at the thought. But I had temporarily put my fears on hold when a nurse friend assured me I was too young to have the disease.

The doctor told me they would run further tests and do an MRI to make sure they had found everything.

I said, "You're looking for Wilson's Disease aren't you. It has some of the same symptoms."

"How do you know about Wilson's Disease?" the doctor asked.

I responded, "Lately I've become very interested in neurological problems. Can you blame me?"

From his reaction, I realized I'd gone far enough with my complaints and over-dramatization. In the meekest of voices I said hopefully, "Isn't it possible that I've just gone crazy? Couldn't that be the cause of my problem?

The doctor answered quickly and firmly, "No, Alice, you are not crazy." He then asked if I wanted treatment.

"Yes, I do."

His next question surprised me. Did I want something that was mentally confusing or something that wasn't mentally confusing?

I returned to my sarcastic mode. "Well, why don't we start with something that's not mentally confusing?"

He then handed me a sample medication and a prescription for Eldepryl, purported to be a fabulous breakthrough in the treatment of Parkinson's, slowing the progression of the disease by 50 percent.

I left the doctor's office in shock. Everything seemed unreal and dreamlike. Looking back, I realize how fortunate I was to get the news so quickly and efficiently. I have read about people who went from doctor to doctor for what seemed like ages before they knew what was wrong with them.

The lab technician was certainly ready to cheer up the sick. The instant she heard that my preliminary diagnosis was Parkinson's and I had expressed my fear of becoming a burden on my wonderful husband, Miss Sunshine offered her own tale of woe.

She'd been a dentist on the East Coast, she said. But, because of her father's decline due to Parkinson's, she'd been forced to give up her practice and move to Washington State to help care for him.

It was time for me to return to work and face my boss and co-workers, who were waiting to hear the doctor's diagnosis. Somehow I managed to drive across the Lake Washington floating bridge to the place where I had been an accountant the past five years, Olympic Jewelers Ltd. of Seattle.

I parked on the street. Ignoring the crosswalk and a van bearing down on me, I headed straight to the store. I was both surprised and embarrassed when the van driver stopped abruptly. He got out and said, "Lady, you just walked in front of my van! There's a crosswalk over there." He pointed in the direction of the crosswalk.

Realizing how irrational I'd been, I turned to him and said sweetly, "You are entirely right, sir, I've behaved stupidly." Robbed of a comeback, he headed back to the van without a word, just a shrug that said, "What's with you, lady?"

The moment I entered the store, Kathy, a co-worker, and Jizel, the boss's daughter, descended on me to ask what the doctor had diagnosed.

"Later," I said, brushing them off.

Jizel said, "Alice, you tell us right now. What's the matter?"

I replied, still unwilling to face the truth head on, "It's bad. It's either a brain tumor or Parkinson's."

Edward, my boss, broke in. "Go home, Alice, right now. We'll see you tomorrow."

I managed to re-cross the street without incident and drove back over the bridge to our lovely Kirkland home.

Although I felt God was with me for the long fight ahead, I was definitely uneasy. When you come from a certifiably nutty family, as I most certainly did, a brain problem of any kind is not high on one's list of preferred diseases.

Chapter Three

WHERE DID THAT
REDHEAD COME FROM?

The day I was born was my mother's own "Doomsday." Before I came along, my mother, born Beulah Smith, had lived a successful and satisfying life. She had graduated from Walla Walla College, a small Seventh-day Adventist school in the southeast corner of Washington State, where she majored in home economics. After college, she met and married my father, Emery Shumate, who was 17 years older than she. They had already welcomed my brother, Victor, into their home. He was two years old when I threw everything out of kilter.

I was born August 18, 1947 in a small hospital in Kirkland, Washington, one of several picturesque little towns on the shores of Lake Washington, east of Seattle. I was formally christened Alice Shumate. It would have been great to hear how excited and happy everyone was that I had joined the family. But, sadly for my mother, such was not the case. Poor Mom was so traumatized she had no recollection of my birth. Something obviously snapped deep within her mind. Crazy as it sounds, because of her reaction the man I would someday marry could have become my brother.

As if my birth weren't enough for Mom to bear, she and my father had chosen that time to move from their beautiful home in Kirkland to a wooded, 140-acre spread outside North Bend, in the foothills of Washington State's Cascade Mountain Range.

My father decided he would build our house this time. He started with the garage, in which we would live while he worked on the main house. Meanwhile, Mom would try to be the perfect home economist without so much as indoor plumbing.

Mom lost it. Today we might quickly recognize her symptoms as post-partum depression, which in its most serious manifestation led Andrea Yates to drown her five children a few years ago. Fortunately Mom's depression didn't lead her to harm her children, but it did grow increasingly worse until she had a classic case of post-partum psychosis.

Dad was not one to quickly recognize a medical emergency. By the time he realized Mom needed treatment she was almost beyond help.

Aunts and uncles were summoned from both sides of the family. All were shocked to find Mom disheveled and totally out of it. They decided that Dad's three sisters should take turns caring for my brother and me. Two of my mother's three brothers chipped in to pay for her to go to a private hospital.

At the hospital Mom was given a series of electric shock treatments. The therapy brought about an initial improvement in her condition, but nothing lasting. Finally the doctors told my Dad and my Aunt Mildred (the capable Irish wife of my mother's eldest brother) that since there probably was no hope of a positive outcome, Mom should be committed to a mental institution.

While Aunt Mildred and Dad drove Mom to the state mental hospital in Steilacoom, southwest of Tacoma, she cheerfully told them she had just discovered how to control the traffic lights. She could do this, she said, by blinking her eyes. One blink would turn the light green, two would turn it red. That demonstration erased all doubt that Mom had to be committed.

What followed next is true, even though it seems unbelievable.

Adaline Crooker, a resident of the valley and a member of the church my folks attended, heard about our family's dilemma. She and her husband had one son, David, and wanted to have more children. Unfortunately, she had miscarried repeatedly. Her solution, since my mother seemed doomed to spend the rest of her life in a mental institution, was to adopt me.

Mrs. Crooker moved David out of his crib and put me in it. I had been in my "new home" only a few weeks when doctors at the state hospital said they wanted Mom to undergo what was then being touted as a "miracle cure" for the insane, the now infamous "ice-pick surgery" or trans-orbital lobotomy.

When Mrs. Crooker heard this, she said, "Take Alice away right now. If I can't have her, I don't want to become attached to her."

Thank heaven my aunts were quick to retrieve me, because many years later her son, David, and I fell in love and married, and as of 2006, we've been married 39 years.

I know there is a God in heaven because He saved my mother. The doctors were enthusiastic about their surgical plans and were energetically rounding up guinea pigs. The doctor who devised the horrific trans-orbital lobotomy had first tried it on corpses. Since corpses do not complain or bring lawsuits, the operation quickly became "standard procedure" for relieving anxiety.

Aunt Mildred was thrilled at the prospect of a cure for Mom and started to work on Dad, who was skeptical of the procedure. With what is known today, he had every right to be.

23

Finally, when it seemed things could get no worse with Mom, he consented to the surgery.

Miracle of miracles, there was immediate improvement in Mom after the operation. Despite the negative effects it had on countless other patients, it was a life-saver for her.

Mom was soon out of the state institution, restored to her intelligent, sane self and my brother and I returned to our home and to her care. The only problem was that she was very perplexed by me. She remembered me as a cute little black-haired baby, and now I was a gangly, redheaded two-year-old who didn't talk.

She badgered my aunts with questions concerning my inability to speak. My aunts responded that I knew how to talk but had quit talking when I was bounced from home to home during my mother's illness. They assured her I would talk when I once again felt comfortable with my family.

My mother continued to worry, chattering away to me about anything and everything in hopes of getting me to respond. Jabbering away as usual one evening, she asked, "What shall we have for dinner tonight?"

Suddenly I blurted, "Pie!" She laughed and laughed with surprise and relief. Her joy must have encouraged me, because she claimed that once I started talking there was no stopping me.

As far as what should be eaten for dinner, pie still sounds good to me. Often I will begin, rather than end, my dinner with dessert. I always say that if someone is going to choke to death it should be on something tasty.

It has been said that one must walk a mile in another person's moccasins to fully understand why that individual reacts to things in a certain way. Being afflicted with

Parkinson's disease and writing this book have opened my eyes to my Mother's situation.

I was never able to understand or really "click" with her. Now I can see why. Most people would have been destroyed by the radical treatment she received. She somehow managed to overcome it. For the rest of her life there was never a dull moment with Mom around.

Chapter Four

LIVING THE HEALTHY LIFE

My family was a collection of unusual people. In most ways, they were remarkable and wonderful and I am thankful to have known and loved them.

As I mentioned before, Mom was a teacher and a perfectionist, a super-motivated, intelligent workaholic. She was busy all the time – teaching school, going to school or working on the house. When she did something, it was done right. She never rested or relaxed and didn't allow me to rest or relax either. Every moment of a person's life, she figured, had to be devoted to something worthwhile.

One day, when she was in the next room, she shouted, "Alice, tell me exactly what are you doing at this moment?" When I replied, straight-faced, "I'm scratching my head," my grandmother, who was in the room, burst into laughter. My mother saw nothing to laugh about.

Whereas my Dad was a "Rare Genius," because he always remembered and never even for an instant forgot I was a special gift from heaven, my Mom never forgot the catastrophic depression my birth had triggered. Dad was an uneducated logger. But he was a shrewd businessperson who ran his own logging operations and did his own accounting. He was unconcerned with the niceties of *House Beautiful*. Much to my mother's consternation, he stored truck tires in the corner of our living room. To him, it was the logical and practical thing to do. They could be stolen from the garage.

We were anything but an ordinary family. In the '50s, the television show *Father Knows Best* typified what passed for the ideal American family, even though most people realized it was fiction. Our family, however, could not benefit from the wisdom dispensed by Robert Young, courtesy of talented scriptwriters. We didn't own a television set.

Television was the least of the luxuries we didn't have. We also didn't have running water in our house. Dad was always digging wells, and those holes in the ground never produced enough water to justify a permanent hookup to the house. Although my big brother spent his childhood hauling water to the house in buckets, we never seemed to have enough water.

One thing we definitely did not have in our home was "evil," as defined by my father. The first thing Dad did with the Sunday paper was open it up, extract the comics and thrust them into the woodstove. He did this to protect our minds from what he considered "senseless pollution."

Dad's fear of pollution from the outside world extended to the types of music we could listen to. Music must be wholesome above all. Mitch Miller's bland music was on the small "approved list" until my father saw Miller's photograph on the cover of a record album. Good grief, the man wore a goatee. Henceforth, there would be no Mitch Miller in our home.

Nor did our family put much faith in the medical profession. Mom had a pretty good reason for being skeptical. Only the grace of God had saved her from a horrendous outcome when doctors performed a lobotomy on her. Defying the odds, she went out post-lobotomy and earned two more college degrees, (from the University of Washington no less) to go with the one she had before the operation.

My folks were fanatical about living in a healthful manner. We were vegetarians – common enough today, but an oddity in the 1950s. Tea and coffee were forbidden—so were cheese and butter. Health was a major part of our religion.

Living in the country, as we did, gave Vic and me freedom to roam 140 acres of woodland, swamp, mountain and rock. We had what many today would call a "perfect environment." Our nearest neighbors were a quarter-of-a-mile down the road. And they were blocked from view by trees, vegetation and a formidable hill.

Mamie Ophelia Smith, my maternal grandmother, spent every summer looking after my brother and me. I use the words "looking after" quite loosely, because grandma was legally blind. The cause of her blindness was no mystery and not uncommon. She had cataracts. Doctors said they could easily remove the cataracts and restore her sight. She didn't believe them.

On the other hand, Grandma had an abiding faith in quacks of all kinds. Every time some hare-brained idea came along, Grandma was a willing guinea pig. Oh, how the scam artists must have loved her. I'll never forget the "ozone machine," which was supposed to restore her sight and cure most ailments known to mankind. The machine did nothing for grandma, but the odor it gave off is unforgettable to this day.

Grandma traveled to Los Angeles for a copper cure, which consisted of attaching her feet to copper plates with wires running to her hands. How this was supposed to improve her eyesight was never clear. When all the "cures" failed, Grandma prayed for divine healing.

Despite her quirks, Grandma was a delightful person, who helped me develop what little patience I now possess. She wrote poetry based on Biblical themes. Her system went like this: I, who could see, would read (over and over and then over again) aloud from the Bible – say, the book of Esther – and Grandma would then compose a poem about it. Then came the tricky part – she did her own typing. Since she couldn't see the keys on a typewriter, I would tell her if her finger was on the right key and she typed away with painful slowness. I loved Grandma, but disliked the typing sessions. It would have been so much simpler if I had simply typed the words for her as she spoke them. But she wouldn't hear of it.

Grandma told me wonderful stories about the family and she had an infectious laugh. She had been a teacher and always paid close, and I mean close, attention to grammar. At church, if a speaker made a grammatical error, the pew would shake with her silent laughter.

Dad's attempts at healthful living were simple. He avoided chocolate as well as most vegetables, went to bed early, arose early and worked, and worked, and then worked some more. He was a thin man and didn't have an extra ounce of weight on his six-foot frame.

A devout believer in warmth, Dad spent an inordinate amount of time making sure my brother and I were warm enough. To assure we didn't get a chill, he stoked the woodstove to capacity during the day and got up in the middle of the night to be sure my brother and I were fully covered by blankets. He insisted that I wear the short version of long-underwear in the wintertime. He also made me wear long cotton stockings. I always said my winter wear made me look like "little old granny piddle pooh."

Mom spent so much time and energy telling me what to eat and when to eat it that it was amazing she had time to get anything done. I was never allowed to eat in peace. And, of course, everything I ate was wrong. If I ate a slice of bread and removed the crust, I was wrong. Even though my plate was full of what she cooked and rationed out to me, I never ate the foods in the right sequence. I often had to sit at the table long after everyone else was through, so I could eat what I didn't want to eat. Many times when no one was looking, I'd load my mouth with food, go outside and spit it under the house.

Every meal with Mom around was a major ordeal. She would start the day with porridge. The mush was bad enough, but worse yet she sometimes added dates and raisins to it. I wanted Cheerios.

My brother joined my mother in the proper eating regime and won her heart by being able to eat and totally enjoy all the things I detested.

What I most hated was peas, which I was forced to eat over my loud protests. I'm quite certain peas will someday be linked to every known disease and be found to be behind most natural disasters. I am certain peas should have warning labels on them. It's logical. The first letter in "peas" is the same one that begins the word "poison".

Since I hated peas, it was only natural Mom should love them. She would pile my plate high with that detestable vegetable. Then she would inform me there would be no dessert unless I ate every spoonful. If I decided I'd win the battle by forgoing dessert, Mom would say menacingly, "Alice, you have five minutes to eat all those peas OR ELSE!"

Failure to finish in the allotted time invariably meant a spanking. Since Mom usually used a willow switch on bare legs to get her point across, and since I was a child who did not like pain, I ate the peas.

The eating battles in our home were long and never-ending. When I was 12, I committed the crime of opening the refrigerator door and eating a tiny sliver of cake. I had just returned from a Valentine's party and Mom was so horrified by this assault on my health that she grabbed Dad's razor strop and whacked me on the rear. I was so offended and angry that I blurted, "I can't wait to get away from here, to where you can't beat me anymore."

Mom's response was predictable. "Bend over," she said. "I'll have to whip you some more, because that's certainly no way to talk to your mother."

I turned into a sneak. During recess at school I'd ask permission to go to town. I'd stop off at the local bakery and pick up a baker's dozen of delicious fresh doughnuts, eating every one (all 13) of them before the day was over. Amazingly, I remained stick-thin.

By the time I was 14, I still had not made much headway with Mom's dietary rules. One Sunday morning I arrived in the kitchen to find that my breakfast consisted of a cereal bowl filled with wheat germ and milk. When I protested that I had no intention of eating such a ridiculous breakfast, my mother issued another of her edicts: eat the wheat germ or spend the entire day in bed. As usual, I wound up following her wishes.

Mom and Dad were as different from each other as iced-tea and hot chocolate. Although she was very quick tempered, Mom never screeched or ranted. In fact, she would never admit she was upset. Dad, on the other hand, was a patient, slow-to-anger type. But, when finally provoked, he made no attempt to hide his wrath. He would roar, "I have had it! I am going to Alaska." After slamming the back door so hard it almost fell off its hinges, he would stride down the driveway with great determination, only to turn around and return to the front yard before heading off again. Dad never made it to Alaska, but he did manage to rid himself of whatever had upset him.

I took after Dad in many ways, acquiring his fiery mannerisms. From Mom, I inherited a short fuse. Even lay people know short fuses and fiery responses are not the road to perfect health. Mom tried to help me in every way, going so far as to tell me about the calm, peaceable, saintly people on her side of the family. They would never, she said, dream of losing their cool under the most trying circumstances.

There was the heart-warming story of "Horace and His Father:"

Horace and his extremely patient father had just pulled into their lovely farmyard in their horse and buggy. Horace's father left the rig, the better to direct his son's parking efforts. In the process, several-hundred pounds of buggy wheel ended up on top of the father's foot. Did that saintly gentleman shriek and yell, as many men might? No, he did not! Remaining calm and collected, even dignified, he said in a quiet voice, "Horace, when you pulled up, you parked the buggy on top of my foot. Please pull up a bit farther." Horace replied, "All right, father; just wait until I can get hold of the reins."

Even our animals were supposed to be good for our health. Dad loved dogs and was highly suspicious of cats. When I asked for a cat, Dad said they were sneaky animals and no good as pets. I later learned his aversion to them had come from his mother because she said they were known to suck the breath

33

from babies in their cribs. Despite the dire warning, I continued to yearn for a cat.

One morning my dream came true. Our dog, who hated cats, had chased one up a tree. It was a large and beautiful cat – one of the prettiest I'd ever seen – although it made nasty hissing noises and glared at my brother and me and at our dog while it was up the tree. We called on Dad to help us rescue the "kitty." Dad took one look at the creature and announced that "kitty" was a bobcat and definitely did not qualify as a household pet. The experience, however, may have softened him. After a few years, he finally allowed us to have a kitten – a gift from a dear family friend.

Some months later, the cat began to behave in a strange manner, rolling around on the floor and making odd noises. Dad beseeched me to call a vet and describe the symptoms to him. The vet laughed and said our cat would soon be having kittens. To avoid any such problems in the future, Dad took all the kittens to the vet and asked which ones were males. Dad then took the mother and the girl cats to the Humane Society and brought home the two boy cats. One of the "boys" was run over by a car – the other had kittens.

In retrospect, it is sad that every child in the world could not have been treated as fairly and kindly as our folks reacted to us on the day we goofed and put our wiggly, waggily black cocker spaniel in the family car. Our neighbor was tired of Skippy. He was sick of Skippy chasing his milk cows and told us in no uncertain terms that he had had it. If he caught Skippy worrying his cows again, he would shoot him. Where we went, Skippy went also. We were going to play with the neighbor's children and Skippy wanted to come. Mom and Dad had held him back, but obviously not long enough because he caught our trail.

We tried everything, but he would not turn back. We knew if he saw the neighbor's cows, he would go for them and were deathly afraid the neighbor would kill him. We spied the car. It had been left at the bottom of the hill because of ice the night before, and we quickly decided it was the answer for everything. We opened the door and Skippy jumped right in. He looked so happy, we thought goody gumdrops! We rolled down the window a bit and ran to the neighbor's house and had a great time with the kids.

On the way home, we stopped by the car to retrieve Skippy and imagine our shock to see that he had torn the entire interior of the car to shreds. He had dug the rug to the floorboards. The front and back seats were history; he had even tried to launch himself through the roof of the car and in the process had pulled down the lining. We did not want to go home. We talked and thought it might be wise to say an awful robber had torn the car up, but decided our parents would probably wonder why the robber didn't just steal the car, so we told the truth. Our parents were so fair and decent. They did not even get mad at us, they simply put the car back together and life went on.

If early influences were the sole determining factor in the outcome of a person's life, then, perfection should have been realized in me. I knew how to be honest, never to spend a penny unnecessarily, how to walk, talk and certainly what and when to eat. Unfortunately it is not always what a person sows that they reap. I am glad my folks never knew the health challenges I faced. Both of them went to rest while my health was still excellent.

There were a few flaws in my family's health system. Truly healthy families relax and take a vacation. Mom and Dad just went on working. I remember them spending one Christmas Eve laying linoleum on the kitchen floor.

When Mom decided to drive Grandma from Washington State to Wisconsin to see her elderly sisters, Dad stayed home to work. As we pulled out of the driveway in the old family Buick, Dad stood and waved goodbye with the saddest look on his face, almost as if he thought he'd never see us again.

The old car's motor first chugged to a halt near Moses Lake, in Eastern Washington. My brother, who was 14 at the time, attempted to fix it. The repair lasted for only a few miles. The only solution was for my brother and me to become human "tow trucks," pushing or pulling the car during its periodic breakdowns until the motor started again. This went on all the way to Wisconsin and back again. I'm sure we set some kind of record for human endurance.

Grandma felt carsick when we were in the mountains and upchucked her healthful breakfast. Mom stopped driving and said, "We will now clean the car." She started cleaning the trunk, my brother disappeared into the woods, and Grandma and I were the only ones not doing anything. So I got busy and cleaned up the mess.

It was on this trip that I was introduced to date sandwiches. One was more than enough for me. I am thankful Mom did not become as fond of date sandwiches as she was of peas.

Although doctors continued to be suspect in our family, they were always called upon after all else had failed. And they generally met the challenge heroically. Such as the time Mom and Dad were out in the woods logging. Vic was in Vietnam and I was in college, so we were no help. Mom was driving the family tractor and Dad was on the truck directing her as she placed logs in the truck bed. Suddenly, a log swung around and crushed Dad against the side of his truck.

Mom leaped from the truck, thrilled to hear that Dad was at least conscious enough to say, "Get that log out of the air, then help me into the truck and drive me home." Mom negotiated the bumpy road with her load of logs and then helped Dad into the house and into bed.

As a precaution, Mom finally called a doctor and calmly asked if she should bring her husband into the office sometime the next day, after she had finished teaching school, "just in case something might be broken." Based on her low-key recitation of Dad's condition, the doctor thought that bringing Dad in the next day would be a good idea.

After serving Dad some hot soup, which he couldn't keep down, Mom began to have second thoughts. Maybe he was worse off than she'd thought. Fortunately, Dad cut her worries short when he said, "I need to go to the hospital, and I had better go right now."

Calling an aid car would be far too theatrical for my parents. Instead, they called the church pastor and my boyfriend, Dave to help Dad walk to the car. After riding to the hospital, Dad got out of the car and walked into the emergency room. Doctors were quick to give him morphine, which he protested was a "bit extreme," before beginning x-rays. The verdict? His pelvis was broken in two places, and he was bleeding internally. He would not have lived through the night if he had stayed home.

Dad and I arrived home simultaneously. He had just been released from rehab and I was on a college break. I will never forget how impressed I was to see Dad hop through the door on his crutches. He was smiling from ear to ear. Later that night he thanked God for the many wonderful blessings He had bestowed on our family.

I wondered at the time what blessings he was being thankful for, since everything seemed bleak to me. My brother was in Vietnam. Dad was unable to work and, being self-insured, he was going to have to pay every medical bill himself.

My folks would earn an F- grade when it came to summoning medical help in a prompt manner. But I would have to give them an A for attitude, effort and good intentions and for being genuinely good people.

Chapter Five

MY BROTHER'S KEEPER

It is not easy for me to write about my brother Victor. I am almost at a loss for words when I try to describe what he did and what might have prompted him to do it.

Victor, who preceded me into the world by two years, was a willful toddler by the time we began our rounds of aunts, uncles and cousins who cared for us while Mom underwent treatment for a mental breakdown.

My earliest memories of Vic can be summed up in a single word: T-R-O-U-B-L-E. Vic was a super-strong-willed child who seemed to be in trouble from the time he got up in the morning until he went to bed at night.

It didn't help that Mom and Dad were authoritarian parents who, rather than give us choices, demanded total compliance with whatever they wanted us to do. I learned early in life not to cross them. Vic, on the other hand, challenged them until little disagreements escalated into full-blown battles.

Spankings were certainly not the answer or remedy for his behavioral problems, but our parents lacked imagination and simply figured if the first one did not work, they would repeat the procedure. I don't know how he did it, but he seemed to gain strength from a spanking and be even more intent on having his own way.

If I could think of a way to avoid being spanked, I availed myself of it. Pain has never held an attraction for me.

Mom decided to keep Vic out of school and teach his first-grade lessons herself. It was a disaster. Vic refused to cooperate. The more he resisted, the more Mom persisted!

For some reason, Mom decided Vic should become a doctor. With her ingrained distrust of the medical profession, it was something I could never understand. Naturally, Vic fought her every inch of the way. She, being equally strong-willed, fought back. Her solution: take Vic to a doctor so he could see how wonderful doctors are.

While the doctor was giving Vic a physical examination, Vic gouged him with his fingernails. After that, whenever Vic heard the word "doctor" he would begin yelling at the top of his lungs.

When Vic was not in trouble or performing his daily chores, which consisted of hauling water and wood to the house, he and I would play. Vic taught me to climb to the top shelves of our cupboards and closets, where I could snoop to my heart's content. During one of our picnics in the woods, I ate skunk cabbage and found it to be anything but tasty. In the summer, we swam in the pond on our property and ventured down into our water well. It was a good thing our parents never found out what we were up to.

At night, when we were in bed but not yet ready to sleep, Vic would whisper from his room across the hall, "Do you want to play SNEAK?"

I, of course, would whisper "Yes," and we'd tiptoe down the hall and creep toward the kitchen to spy on Mom and Dad.

At parochial school, where grades 1-8 were in a single classroom, Vic's antics drove the teachers to distraction but won the hearts of his fellow students. One day we had a substitute teacher and Vic decided to stage a special performance. Wearying of Vic's antics, the teacher relegated him to a side room, apart from the rest of the class.

To gain attention, Vic inserted a string through the keyhole. In a loud voice, he informed the class and the substitute teacher that when the string began to move he would begin a special broadcast. Sure enough, the string moved when he pulled on it, and he began to sing in a loud voice and jabber all sorts of goofy things. The class loved it, until our church pastor walked in the door – a signal that the party was over.

Vic could be wildly entertaining. He would take Grandma's cane and balance it on his nose. He could stand on his head and walk on his hands. He once walked half-a-mile in dog fashion, with boots on his hands.

When it came time for high school, Vic was sent to a private boarding school near the town of Auburn, about an hour's drive from our home. He got into trouble almost immediately and, after spring break, was suspended from school for the rest of the year. He returned to the school the next year and I went with him. This time he managed to stay in school with no trouble. He was a great help to me because he had a knack for hanging on to money. After I had spent mine, I would hit Vic up for a loan. He never failed me.

Unfortunately, Vic never did catch up on the studies he missed that first year. When it came time to graduate, he was not among those who earned a diploma and he never returned to school.

Mom and Dad never gave up on Vic. They harped on how important education was and why it was imperative that he return to school. Of course, the more they hounded the more Vic resisted.

Vic got a job as a construction worker, earning a reputation as hard-working and reliable. He had a girlfriend, Rosie, with whom I worked in a nursing home during the summer. Despite the heavy lifting, we had a good time.

Dave often visited Vic, and we became acquainted. Before long, Vic, Rosie, Dave and I were going out together on weekends.

When the Vietnam War came along, Vic was a prime candidate for active duty. He was unmarried, no longer in school and not employed in a "critical" occupation. Our family was heartsick when his draft notice arrived in the mail. We were terrified of losing him.

Vic declared himself a conscientious objector, opposed to guns but willing to serve as a medic. He trained at Fort Sam Houston, Texas, and left for Vietnam while I was in college. He served as a litter-bearer with the 93rd Evacuation Hospital, near Saigon, running to helicopters when they landed and bringing the wounded to the hospital as quickly as possible. When larger planes landed, he and other litter-bearers unloaded the bodies and body parts of those who had died in the war.

After a year in Vietnam, Vic was sent back to Fort Ord, California, to finish his Army service. Like a lot of young men who served in that war, Vic returned to us in body but not in mind.

While Vic was gone, Dave and I decided we wanted to be married and became engaged in July, 1966, one month before he was called into the service. One year later, we were married. Vic came up for the wedding and we talked and played some of our old table games. I didn't see anything wrong with him at the time. A few days after the wedding, Dave and I flew to Fort Detrick, Maryland, where Dave was to be stationed for the next year. While we were there, Vic married Rosie.

Upon Dave's discharge and our return to Washington State, we noticed that Vic had taken to ranting and raving constantly about the Communists being the cause of the world's problems. Vic had always been high-strung, of course, and we rationalized his ravings as a natural winding down from his bloody experiences in Vietnam. Had we been really alert, we would have sought medical attention.

Vic's ranting began focusing on numerous "conspiracies" he believed were taking over the country. To the Communists, he added Jews, the Rockefeller family and, finally, sugar. You know, the sweet stuff many of us crave. Vic collected reams of material on these "conspiracies," and he would prattle on interminably, until we were totally fed up with hearing him.

Vic's behavior became increasingly bizarre. He took Rosie's washing machine apart and left it in pieces on the floor because, he said, he had more important things to do than put it back together. The "important things" were nonstop ranting and raving.

Things came to a head with the premature birth of Vic and Rosie's beautiful daughter, Kimberly. Vic, who had recently fallen prey to some serious eating hang-ups, decided that Kim – who weighed a scant four pounds at birth – should be fed every four hours, on the dot. Kim would be hungry and cry, but if it wasn't her rigidly scheduled feeding time, there would be no food and she would simply cry herself to sleep. Kim would have become skin and bones if Rosie had allowed Vic to have his way. Fortunately, deciding she'd had enough of Vic's nuttiness, she filed for divorce. Vic was devastated, and in time Rosie relented and took him back. Although she did her best to make things work, Vic's screwball behavior eventually developed into full-blown meanness and violence.

After the final breakup of their marriage, Vic lost what had remained of his sense of humor. His mission in life was to tell everyone what and when to eat. The "ill-effects of sugar" consumed him. He would preach loudly on the subject for hours on end. It was exhausting to be in the same room with him.

One Thanksgiving I tried to appease Vic by serving a sugarless meal. It was a tasteless and gloomy affair, not the least bit festive. While I was trying to get my kitchen back to normal after the dinner, Vic appeared at my side and started nagging me about having sugar in my cupboard. I finally lost it and said, "Shut up!"

As Vic spiraled out of control, he turned totally against eating, lecturing us on the wonders of fasting. He also turned against Christmas, birthdays and almost everything else that people enjoy.

Sometimes he'd come to our house and sleep on the floor. When Dave was at work and I was busy cleaning the house and washing clothes, Vic would follow me everywhere I went, ranting all the while about how worthless women were. For some odd reason, I was unable to appreciate or sympathize with his viewpoints.

When he was not at our house, he would visit Mom and Dad and boss them around. The only good times were when Vic got a job driving a logging truck and couldn't spend full-time bothering us.

Rosie requested and was granted child support in the divorce decree. Vic refused to pay, despite our arguments that he had fathered Kim and was responsible for her. Vic was too busy telling us how to live our lives to listen to anything we had to say.

One day, Dad fell in the yard and broke his hip.

Poor Dad, if only Vic and Mom had called an aid car, or failing that, if only they had put Dad in the car and driven him to a hospital. But, between Vic and Mom – Vic insisting against all evidence that Dad would be all right and Mom failing to overrule him – Dad, who should have lived to be at least 95, was doomed.

When Dad finally was lifted to his feet, Vic decided that what his father needed most was exercise. That's right, exercise on a broken hip. Mom's contribution was to decide that Dad needed a shower. Meanwhile, poor Dad continued to complain of hip pain.

By the time Mom called to ask me what she should do, I told her to call a doctor immediately, because if Dad had trouble walking something was seriously wrong. She said Vic, the trained medic, was opposed to calling a doctor.

Dave and I went to see Dad and were horrified at his condition. We begged Mom to call a doctor. Still she refused. When we got home, I got on the phone to Mom and, for the first time in my 37 years on planet Earth, I screamed at her: "For the love of Pete, you had better call a doctor."

Mom was shocked. But did she heed my advice? Of course not. She said she was terribly upset at my behavior, that she had spent her entire life wondering if I would someday have a nervous breakdown. Now, considering the way I had screamed at her, it was obvious that her worst fears had been realized. Talk about denial!

For two weeks Dad remained at home, being treated by two quacks – Mom and Vic. For the record, Dad was also to blame. He had never liked going to a doctor until zero hour.

Finally, when it was far too late, Mom did what she should have done immediately. She called for an aid car. As Dad left the house, Mom looked at him and promised, "I will bring you home." And she should have added, "When you are better."

Dad was beyond help by the time the doctors saw him. His heart was so bad he was in no condition to undergo surgery on his hip. The last time I saw him, he was thin and weak and I spent an hour trying to get him to eat something. I begged Mom to assist him in his eating and to get volunteer help if necessary.

Nothing I said mattered in the least. I had only taken one-half of the nurse's training BS degree at Walla Walla College and was on the side of sense and sanity. Why listen to me?

I kept in constant touch with the hospital staff concerning Dad's condition and care and was as shocked and outraged as they were when I learned that Mom was checking Dad out of the hospital.

I asked the hospital staff, "What's the plan here – to have him croak at home?"

A staff member replied that it was obvious my mother wanted just that.

When I inquired about a daughter's legal right in such matters, I was informed that I had none. But they did advise me to talk to the doctor and to my mother.

In fairness to Mom, Dad repeatedly spoke just one word: "Home."

The doctor said that not only was Mom determined to take Dad home, but he felt that while her natural remedies wouldn't cure Dad, they probably wouldn't hasten his death. He made no mention of the fact that Mom was a 105-pound bundle of rheumatoid arthritis and totally unable to move Dad around. Instead, he added, "Your father is 82 years old and a bit hard of hearing."

I retorted, "He still enjoys shopping and he happens to be my Dad and I like him, so how about that?"

The doctor informed me that he was not God, which I already knew.

Next I called Mom and tried to reason with her. "Why move Dad at this stage? How can you possibly care for him?"

Mom reacted like a desperate, cornered animal. She said, "Alice, if you do anything to throw a monkey wrench in my plans, I will never speak to you again as long as I live."

I was surprised and hurt by her words and wished we could work together in a reasonable manner.

I made a quick decision. Dad was going to die if we left him in the hospital. If we took him home, he also would die. I might as well let Mom do as she wished, because the result would be the same.

An ambulance took Dad on his final trip home. The next morning, the telephone rang. It was Mom. It was with a sense of relief that I heard the words: "Daddy's gone."

The "Rare Genius" was gone! I realize there is a time to be born and a time to die, that nobody lives forever. But it would have been easier for me to accept the loss of my father – who had always been my buddy, with never a cross word – if Mom and Vic had done everything possible to help him on the day he fell in the yard.

I am still amazed that my mother, who refused to listen to anything I had to say while Dad was alive, left me to handle most of the arrangements after he was gone. When there were decisions to make at the funeral home, she simply closed her eyes and let me decide. Until it came time to choose a coffin, that is.

Because Dad had been a logger and had driven logging trucks, I wanted him to have a beautiful wooden coffin. Mom wanted a metal one, "because his truck was metal and that makes sense." I was glad to welcome her back to the world of decisions and planning.

While we were making these decisions, Mom suddenly was overwhelmed with the notion that she must see Dad right then. No waiting. "You don't want to see him now," the funeral director said. "He has no clothes on. We are working on him. You won't like what you see."

Mom didn't care what he looked like. She wanted to see him right now. Finally, the people at the funeral home put her off by saying that Dad's body was down with other bodies and he simply could not be seen at that time. But they promised to get him ready soon.

As for me, I was in no hurry to see him. Looking at people who have died has never brought me joy, peace or closure. When we finally saw Dad, I wasn't happy with the way his mouth looked. But I wasn't happy with much of anything right then. People fall and break their hips often. That's one of the reasons we have aid cars, hospitals, doctors, nurses and painkillers. Dad was denied these things when they could have helped.

The funeral was scheduled for Saturday, the burial the following Monday. In the company of my husband Dave, my mother-in-law, Adaline, and our children, I arrived at the funeral home for the service. Vic was at the door greeting the mourners.

I was in the family room, waiting for the service to begin, when the funeral director approached and said, "We need to get your brother in here, so we can start the service." Vic, he said, was walking up and down the street, refusing to come into the funeral home.

I got up and headed for the street, where I found Vic pacing back and forth. He looked anguished and unglued. I said,

"Come on Vic, everyone's waiting. We have to get the service started. This is becoming embarrassing."

Vic gave me a guilt-ridden look and said, "Go ahead and start the funeral without me. I told Dad I wouldn't attend his funeral if he died before he was 94 years old. I figure if I come in five minutes late that will be good enough."

I went back inside and told the funeral home people what Vic had said. The service was started without him. Sure, enough, Vic arrived a few minutes later.

When the service ended, I stood by Dad's coffin, taking one final look at his mouth, wishing it looked better. The undertakers approached. One said, "You have to stop your brother."

"Stop him from what?" I said, with a growing sense of horror.

"He wants to take your father home," was the reply.

"Tell him it's against the law," I said.

"It's not against the law, but we are trying to talk your brother into leaving your father here," was the response. "We have promised to put your Dad in a special room, so your brother can stay with him as long as he wants to. But your brother won't settle for that."

"Where's the preacher?" I asked.

I was steered to Pastor Rasmussen, who listened politely to my plea for help. The service had been fine, I said, but I was upset because there would have been no need for a service if my Mom and brother had done the right thing after my Dad fell and broke his hip. And now my crazy brother wanted to take Dad home in his coffin.

Poor Dad, who had always been so dignified, who never liked to be a public spectacle. Why, he had even been reluctant to take me on a roller coaster ride at the Western Washington

Fair, because he was afraid I would scream and call attention to myself and to him. Now he was lying in a coffin and in the middle of a ridiculous family dispute.

Pastor Rasmussen, looking quite angry, headed downstairs to confront Vic. Our family followed. Vic didn't want to listen to reason. When I reminded him that he had a bad back and couldn't possibly move the coffin into the house, he became more determined than ever.

Someone had the presence of mind to ask Vic why on earth he felt he had to take his Dad home in a coffin. His reply was disturbing in what it revealed about his twisted state of mind: "Dad refused to go on a trip to California with me, so I am going to take him home now."

Mom was asked her opinion. She said, "Whatever will make Vic feel better."

At that point, I said, "I have had enough. I am going home." Dave and I, Dave's mother and our children left. We would not be attending the graveside service on Monday.

What happened from that point on is hearsay, but very reliable hearsay.

Vic returned to the mortuary the next morning and took Dad, in his coffin, back to our parents' home in his station wagon. He parked in the carport and spent the night on the ground, alongside the station wagon and the coffin. He likened it to going on a camping trip with Dad.

In time for the graveside service, Vic drove to the cemetery, where he was met by the extremely patient undertakers. They agreed to his request that the coffin be re-opened so he could see Dad once more.

Finally they closed the coffin, confident that Vic was through interfering with their normally smooth-running operation. They were wrong once again. A couple drove up just as the service was about to begin and Vic insisted that the undertakers open the coffin once more so they could view Dad.

To this day, I wonder why Mom and Vic were so quick to let my father die and so slow to allow him to be buried.

With Dad finally in the ground, I thought the nightmare with my family was over. In truth, it was just getting started.

Chapter Six

KEEPING MOM ALIVE

After we lost Dad, Dave and I were so frustrated with Vic and Mom that we decided to take a break from them. We stayed as far away from them as possible. We even drove to California to visit my Aunt and Uncle for Christmas. Shortly after, Dave, a graduate forester, received a promotion from his employer, Burlington Northern Timberlands and we moved from Battleground to Kirkland, Washington.

Vic showed up at our new home one day and launched into justifications for his abnormal behavior after Dad's fall. Doctors, he said, had killed Dad. If only Dad had quit eating, as he wanted him to, he would have recovered from his broken hip. Furthermore, if we all had had enough faith Dad surely would have been brought back to life after the medical profession pronounced him dead.

When Mom turned Dad over to the murderous doctors, he had become so discouraged because he knew that was it—Dad was done for! He had intended to let everything just go and do nothing more, but then he had thought it over and that is when he decided maybe he could do something helpful after all. The "something helpful" was to take Dad home from the funeral service. Dying, he concluded, was the unpardonable sin. The more Vic talked the more I realized he had lost all touch with reality.

Mom and I tried to care for each other during these trying times. But the next nine years were a nightmare as Vic—who had caused Dad nothing but misery—moved in with Mom and devoted all his energy to "keeping Mom alive."

Dave and I were caught squarely in the middle of the war of words and nutty ideas that raged between two health addicts, Mom and Vic.

In a way, Mom was trapped. She knew Vic was mentally ill, but she loved him and didn't realize that the best thing she could do was stay as far away from him as possible.

When Vic was at Mom's home, he nagged her constantly. When Vic was away, Mom worried herself sick over whether he was taking proper care of himself. At such times, she'd call and ask me what she should do.

Vic still wouldn't pay a penny of child support for his daughter. To beat the court system, he would hold a job but refuse to accept any pay from his employer. That way, there wouldn't be any way to get money out of him. A judge ordered Vic to supply the names of 10 employers who had refused to hire him. Vic, as usual, did not comply. He was, after all, working.

Things came to a head when the long arm of the law actually caught him driving the logging truck for a company that had "hired" him. Vic was arrested and committed to the King County jail.

Mom was worried sick, because Vic had recently discovered the joy of eating absolutely nothing. He would go for days subsisting on nothing but air and water. Worse, he tried to get Mom – already very underweight – to join him in this perverted pursuit of good health. Mom was convinced Vic wouldn't eat a thing in jail and she asked me to call the authorities and warn them of his behavior. I did so, saying that

Vic was a Vietnam veteran, mentally ill and almost certainly would stage a hunger strike.

Our worst fears were realized. When Vic was freed, after 32 days in jail, he weighed just 107 pounds. For a man just a shade under 6-feet tall this was ridiculous.

After seeing him, I called the jail and said I wanted to lodge a formal complaint about the way Vic had been treated. The authorities responded by saying that Vic had been interviewed daily by psychiatrists during his stay in jail. He had been diagnosed as having serious mental problems, not helped a bit by his refusal to eat.

I was further informed that it was my duty, as Vic's sister, to see that he got help. Great! The jail system couldn't help Vic, but supposedly I could.

Vic eventually regained some of his lost weight, but he continued to eat very little, and he would go on long fasts. One day I returned home from work to find Vic waiting for me. In his hand was a sheet of mimeographed paper that told about a man living to be 500 years old simply because he had quit eating. Even more astounding, this health nut had grown a new set of teeth. I said, "Well, he didn't do quite as well as Methuselah (reputed to have lived 900 years) now did he?"

Vic would fix on an idea, however illogical, and then he would believe anything that tended to support his belief. One of his favorite stories was about some people who had drilled deep into the earth and found a rock, which they sawed in half. Inside the rock, they found a live frog. And why was that frog alive, inside a rock? Simple; it hadn't eaten anything for centuries.

"Americans," Vic said, "are killing themselves with their forks. If only they would just stop eating." Now, all one has to do is watch people walking on city streets or in a mall to realize there are a tremendous number of overweight and grossly obese people in this country. They simply eat too much. But going to the other extreme, as Vic preached, makes no sense either.

Vic soon added a new wrinkle to his food fixation. Cayenne pepper, he announced, does wonders for one's health and well-being when it is poured into the eyes. And "skunk spray," he declared, gave him a real boost.

If Vic had kept his crazy ideas to himself, we would have had only Vic to worry about. But he wielded great influence over Mom, who was 5 feet 4-1/2 inches tall, weighed barely 100 pounds and had rheumatoid arthritis. Vic continued to pester Mom daily with his latest eating and fasting schemes.

When Mom could stand it no longer, she'd call me and say, "Please commit your brother to an institution." So, I would call the authorities and ask for help, and they would tell me that it was a police matter. I'd tell Mom what I'd been told to do, and she would plead with me not to call the police, because they almost certainly would put Vic back in jail and he couldn't survive another prolonged hunger strike.

I didn't give up and continued to call the mental-health community. "Why are you calling?" I would be asked. "If your brother is 18 years old or older, he is capable of making this call for help by himself." When I asked how many people with mental-health problems are capable of self-diagnosis, I was told that I might have a point. Then they shifted the blame to Mom, saying that if Vic bothered her she should simply not put up with the situation.

When I added still another problem to the equation – telling them that my mother had undergone a trans-orbital lobotomy – they had no response except to offer their final solution: "Lady, if you are bothered by what's happening between your mother and brother, why don't you just go into counseling yourself and learn to live with the problem."

I was told by one mental-health expert that Vic's behavior at Dad's funeral hadn't been bizarre at all. It was perfectly natural that Vic would want to take Dad's coffin home, because that's what they did in Vietnam. And when I, in growing disbelief, related Vic's "frog story," I was told that many rational people believe that story.

I began to have serious doubts about the mental health of some of the mental-health experts.

During the nine years that Mom lived after Dad's death, there was not much peace, especially if Vic was around. Mom escaped him briefly when she went to Delta Junction, Alaska, to fill in for a teacher who was unable to finish the term. It was a great time for us. But then Vic announced he was going to drive to Alaska to bring Mom home when her teaching stint ended.

The trip home was a disaster. Vic wouldn't stop for Mom to eat. He had brought a few cans of beans to tide her over, "heating" the cans by placing them on his car's manifold. Nothing was too good for Mom!

Another reprieve came when Mom got a job teaching the children of missionaries in Hong Kong. When she arrived home after months away from Vic's meddling, she looked 20 years younger.

But soon the health roller-coaster began another bizarre ride. Vic was alarmed that Mom was no longer skin and bones. Add to that his latest fear: People were trying to poison him, and, by extension, his Mom.

We invited Mom to our home for a Mother's Day breakfast. Vic called to beseech me not to poison our mother. I told him to relax; I wouldn't be doing the cooking. That would be done by Dave, and our teenage son, Dan. That did not console him in the least. Vic cautioned me that I also could be a target of poisoning.

After talking to Vic, I realized I could not stand to spend a weekend listening to still another of Vic's tirades about eating. I used to wonder why on earth when there were so many interesting subjects to discuss, all he could think about was eating – it was always about eating. I also wondered why it was never a discussion just a nonstop monologue about sugar. I would often feel an uncontrollable urge to grab about a 10 pound bag of sugar and guzzle it on the spot to see what his reaction would be. Instead, I called and said that instead of having Vic and Mom come to our house for Mother's Day, I would pay them a visit on Saturday afternoon and not interrupt their routine.

When I arrived on Saturday, Vic met me in the front yard and refused to allow me in the house. He said he knew I was trying to have him jailed, and I replied that he was wrong that I wanted to keep him out of jail. If he went to jail he wouldn't eat anything and I didn't want that to happen. I told him my only desire was that he let Mom eat as she wished.

Mom emerged form the house and we drove to a nearby park, where Vic and Mom bickered constantly. Mom said Vic had torn her desk to pieces and poured a jug of water on it because she told him she wanted to eat. Vic said Mom had cursed him. Mom, who never swore, responded that Vic had been operating on her feet with a knife and had refused to stop when she told him to.

My parting advice to Vic that day was this: "Get a life and leave Mom alone to live hers." I asked Mom to come home with me. She said she had to stay to help Vic. I was very upset when I left them.

Vic's mental state seemed to worsen by the day. He would not allow Mom to read anything that didn't have his stamp of approval, and the only things on his approved list were health books. He would force her to sit in the bathtub for three hours at a time. He would not allow her to clean the house. He would take her on long forced marches. He would turn the heat down so low that Mom was half-frozen most of the time. And, of course, because Mom had been diagnosed with cataracts, Vic insisted on his favorite cure for all eye problems: a solution containing cayenne pepper.

Mom called one day to say she thought things were getting better. I didn't ask what in the world had caused her to become hopeful.

Later that week, when I called the house, Vic got on the phone and bragged about his new treatment for Mom. She was on a new diet of cayenne pepper, water, lemon juice and maple syrup. When I asked how long she'd been on that diet, he replied, "Ten days."

I asked that Mom be put on the phone. "How much did she weigh now?"

"Eighty-five pounds," she replied.

I lost it, demanded that she put Vic back on the phone and told him, "This is it! I don't care what you eat, when you eat or where you eat. But this is a free country and if you ever interfere with Mom's eating again, I will call a deputy sheriff."

Vic responded that if I called a deputy sheriff he would disappear and we would never see or hear from him again.

My answer to him was not to threaten me with what he would do, but to think about what I would do.

Mom and I were both worried. Mom was afraid Vic might kill her, or even worse maim her. I thought killing was more likely.

To escape Vic, Mom decided to visit relatives in California over the Christmas holidays. Vic said she shouldn't go. When she insisted, Vic threw all her tomatoes away. It took a call to the sheriff and help from the neighbors to get Mom out of the house.

By this time, it was obvious to all that Mom should never live under the same roof as Vic. We convinced her to let Vic stay in the house, along with the mess he'd created, and find herself a little apartment. She lived with us for a time, then moved in with my gracious, stable father-in-law and mother-in-law.

Her eating habits had become so bad during her time with Vic that she had several episodes with her health. A doctor warned that it was imperative that she eat regularly.

Mom might have lived for a long time, but she couldn't stop worrying about Vic. She talked the in-laws into taking her back to her home. Vic was delighted to see her. But when be started talking about how he was going to bring her back to good health, Mom suddenly decided she didn't want to stay. The in-laws brought her back to our place so she could have enough peace, quiet and food to enable her to plan rationally for the future.

We were happy to take her in. And we decided to deal with her health problems in what, we felt, was a sensible manner. She had cataracts. We allowed her to have cataract surgery. She needed to eat. We let her eat. She needed to see doctors. We allowed her to see doctors. She was only 73, and still quite capable of driving on her own, so we went car shopping with her. Soon she was driving to her doctor's office. We put her in charge of her own health.

Dave and I were thrilled. Everything was going to be fine. We had arranged to go to Switzerland for our 25th wedding anniversary. When we left, Mom agreed to find an apartment and let us know where she was living as soon as we arrived home.

We arrived home to find Mom gone and our worst fears realized. There was no apartment. She had returned to Vic almost as soon as our plane took off. She was apologetic, but felt Vic needed her.

A short time later, a woman friend of Mom's called and said she was concerned. Mom had been trying to leave the house and had asked the woman to find her an apartment. She had found the apartment, but couldn't get any response from Mom.

I called Dave and said, "I'm afraid for Mom. We'd better get down there and see what's happened." We both took a day off from work and went to Mom's place.

We arrived on a cold November day to find Vic stuffing Mom's mouth full of potato peelings. He wouldn't let us in the house. He put a coat on Mom and pushed her out the door, in her stocking feet, to continue her visit with us. We put Mom in the car and drove away quickly.

We stopped at a friend's house to borrow some shoes for Mom. During our trip, we learned that Vic had chopped up her favorite pair of shoes because he was upset that she had undergone cataract surgery instead of being "cured" by his cayenne pepper concoction.

Although the apartment that a friend had found for Mom wasn't quite suitable – no shower, just a bathtub – we scouted around and found an old hospital that had been converted into apartments. It had an elevator and no one could enter the building without a key. Best of all, the landlady promised to keep an eye on Mom.

We went shopping and Mom got a bed and a chest of drawers and arranged to have them delivered to the apartment the next day. We dropped Mom off at her home, so she could pack. Vic wasn't there. She left a note for him the next morning, saying she'd found an apartment.

Vic was so mad he vowed not to speak to me for a year. I would have been happier if it had been more like a thousand years!

You just have to take what you get though.

Dave, the kids and I enjoyed peace for three whole months, from November to February. When Dave turned 50, the kids and I decided to celebrate by taking him to Disneyland. We had a wonderful time. But I returned home to find Mom's telephone disconnected. I knew what that meant—she was back with Vic.

Mom called a few weeks later and told our son she wanted us to come over immediately. We had plans for the evening, so I called the sheriff's department and asked if someone could go to Mom's home and check on her condition. When we got home, I called the sheriff for a report and was told the sheriff's deputies had found the house vacant. They had further learned that my mother had returned to her apartment.

The next morning we called Mom's apartment again and found the phone was now working. We hurried down to see her and get the full story.

It was true that as soon as we had left for Disneyland, Mom had visited Vic and, a charmer when he wanted to be, he had once again talked her into returning to the house. But after a week of Vic's domineering ways, she went to see a doctor, who said she had two options: go into a hospital or go back to her apartment immediately.

Mom decided to return to her apartment. But first she must find a way to escape from Vic. She told him she was going in the car to have her hair done. Vic refused to let her go, saying the hairdresser might poison her. He told her to cancel the appointment. She refused. Vic shook her. She grabbed the phone and called 911. Vic yanked the phone off the wall.

When the deputy arrived, Mom was sitting on the back porch and Vic was fixing her hair. Vic went out to assure the deputy that all was well, but Mom followed him and asked the deputy to please detain Vic long enough for her to leave. The deputy asked why she wanted to leave, and she said Vic wouldn't let her eat and had shaken her.

The deputy said he would arrest Vic and wanted Mom to press charges. When she refused to do so, the deputy said, "Then I'll charge him myself."

End of saga?

Hardly.

Once Vic was jailed, all Mom could think about was his welfare. She called to say she was sure he'd starve. I was in no mood for this. I replied that our daughter, Becky, now a junior in college, was home for her last weekend before leaving for a quarter of study in England. I added, "You know what, Mom, I don't care where Vic is or whether he's eating or not eating. All I want is a few days with absolutely no thought of Vic."

After venting my feelings, I hung up the phone and put in a couple of calls on my own. Vic, I learned, was no longer in jail. He was in Western State Hospital undergoing two weeks of psychiatric evaluation. I called Mom to fill her in on what was happening.

The doctor at Western State was pleased to talk with me and learn our family history. I told him that, frankly, I thought the mental-health experts had failed to diagnose Vic's mental problems in the past and I hoped he'd do better.

He said there not only was no doubt about Vic's mental illness, and he would declare Vic unfit to stand trial for domestic abuse. For once, a doctor did everything he said he would do.

Finally, after years of despair, there was a glimmer of hope that Vic would get the treatment he needed. But my joy was not shared by Mom, who told me she would not sign the commitment papers.

We ended up with a three-way conference call between a social worker, Mom and me. I begged Mom to relent and give Vic a chance at treatment. She steadfastly refused. And I was told that I could not commit Vic because I had not been an eyewitness to what went on. Nor could the deputy sheriff commit Vic.

After Mom left the phone, the social worker told me she thought my mother's inability to deal with Vic's situation stemmed from her trans-orbital lobotomy. She asked if I wanted to appoint a guardian for her. I replied, "No, not as long as she stays away from Vic. She has three college degrees and people respect her and I don't want to undermine that."

But the whole episode clearly demonstrated the frightening reality of mental-health care in my state of Washington, and elsewhere too, I imagine. People in desperate need of help do not get it because the criteria for treatment are so stringent. The rights of the mentally ill are important, of course. But, what about the rights of the relatives of the mentally ill?

Mom came to our home to stay the weekend when Vic's daughter, Kim, graduated from college. While there, Mom dropped another of her bombshells, saying "I'm thinking of moving back with your brother."

"If you do," I replied, "I will commit you. And let me tell you, I won't even have to think twice about it! Enough is enough." I was stressed the whole weekend by her remark and when she was leaving on Sunday, I told her, "Mom, I've been mad at you this entire visit because you said you might be going back with Vic."

Mom smiled sweetly and said she hadn't noticed my displeasure. That was to be Mom's final visit to our home. I wish it had not ended that way.

I was at work when the call came. An emergency room physician told me they had Mom and were keeping her alive on a pacemaker. I was shocked and said, "Do you mean she won't live through the day?" The physician couldn't guarantee it. I told him I was on my way.

God works in mysterious ways. I consider it providential that I missed my bus that morning and drove myself to work. I grabbed the car, got some gas and headed for Centralia, a small town about 85 miles south of Seattle. I was driving about 80 miles an hour on Interstate 5 when I lost power and had to pull to the side of the freeway. I raised the hood of the car and waited for help, which arrived shortly in the form of a Washington State trooper.

The trooper gently asked what the trouble was and I burst into tears. "Everything," I said. "My mother is dying and now my car has quit on me. Furthermore, there's no one to help me. My daughter is in England. My husband and our son are on a canoe trip in Canada. And my brother is crazy. But if I can get to a car-rental place and if a tow truck can take this car to a shop I'll be on my way." The trooper immediately arranged for a tow truck and then drove me to a car-rental outlet.

With my new set of wheels, I arrived at the hospital to find Mom alive but out of it. She kept trying to pull the oxygen mask from her face so she could get out of bed. I stayed by her side, replacing the oxygen mask when she'd yank it off. She didn't seem to recognize me.

65

I was asked if I wanted Mom to be put on a respirator. I said that depended on how much of her mind was left. I was told that nobody could say. Then a doctor called and over the phone assured me that Mom not only could recover completely but could even drive her car again.

Once again the medical profession had left me in a quandary.

The decision was taken out of my hands temporarily when Mom once more pulled off the oxygen mask and I once again put it back on. This time I yelled, "Mom, you need to get better. Your mother lived to be 91, and you have a long way to go. I will be back tomorrow."

Mom responded by setting off every alarm in the place. The emergency crew arrived and asked me to leave the room. While I waited in the hall, I wondered what on earth I was supposed to accomplish. A nurse told me they had stabilized Mom. Then two doctors arrived, one telling me that Mom had suffered enough and I should let her go, the other – a doctor named Fritz – saying I should do everything possible to save her.

I agreed with Dr. Fritz and left for the drive back home. I arrived at about 2 a.m., and the phone rang soon after. It was the hospital staff telling me Mom had been placed on a respirator.

After several days, Dr. Fritz said he was sorry to report that Mom not only wouldn't recover but she could go at anytime. In the meantime, Dave had returned from Canada and we went down to visit her, having been told she would almost certainly die that day.

When we arrived, Mom talked a lot about dying. Dave asked Mom if she was in pain. If not, he said, why don't you just stick around a bit longer. He then handed her some mail. She quickly shuffled through it and saw a check. "Money," she said enthusiastically, "maybe I will live a little longer."

From that moment on, Mom's death was put on hold. She immediately began to improve. She went to rehab, returned to her apartment and drove her car again. We did not have another cross word between us and she told me she was glad to have a second chance at life. She visited Vic but did not attempt to live with him. She made a living will and organized her affairs.

Mom spent a nice summer. And then, on Sept. 3, 1993, an emergency room doctor called me at home to say Mom was at the hospital and this most likely was the end. He told me of her living will and asked if I wanted to override it. I said, "No, but I'm on my way down."

I dressed and drove down to the hospital. Mom was glad to see me and said she was so sick she wanted to die. I told her I was afraid she was going to get her wish this time, adding that I loved her and was going to miss her.

I asked if she wanted me to get Vic. She replied that their last visit had been pleasant and she would let it go at that.

We wrote notes back and forth as her voice became weak. She wanted me to go to her apartment and feed the fish. That evening it was obvious she was slipping and I told her I'd stay the night with her.

In the morning she passed away peacefully. God was very good to me, because I was holding her in my arms at the time, she was in no pain and she had even been trying to eat her breakfast.

I alerted the nurses that Mom was gone and asked them to call the funeral home that had helped us with Dad. But, in truth, I wasn't really sure if they'd want to deal with us a second time.

Dave and Becky came down and the three of us drove over to the old family home, where Vic was now living, to tell him that Mom had died. I pounded on the door repeatedly, but there was no answer. It suddenly dawned on me that this place was now as much mine as it was Vic's and I was curious to see how it looked inside. The signs outside were not promising. A blackberry vine had grown up through the front porch and was making its way through the front door.

The moment I tried to open the door, Vic appeared, giving me a hateful look. I said, "I'm sorry, but I have bad news."

Vic said, "I'll come out." He came out the back door and walked away from me as if he were afraid of what I had to say. I approached him and said, "We lost Mom this morning. She was so sick. I don't think you would have wanted to see her. She told me you had a very pleasant visit the last time you were together. He grabbed me and said, "I forgive you."

The undertakers came and we had another go-round. They knew what to expect from Vic and so did I. Vic put a branch from her apple tree in her casket, "In case she gets hungry and would like a bite to eat.

He had been thinking (this was always very scary) and had decided it was of the utmost importance that we retain a sense of humor and that he had seen a dead snake on the road and thought a good test to see if Mom had really died would be to put the road kill in her coffin. I arranged to have Mom buried before the service so there could be no repeat of Dad's camping trip. Thank Heavens!

I was genuinely pleased to hear of the progress that had come about in Washington State laws concerning burials. It was now mandatory that if a family member wished to do anything out of the ordinary, the rest of the family had to agree. I told the undertakers I would be home and if Vic came up with any bizarre ideas they should call and I would not answer the phone.

We were happy with our plan as that took care of any conflicts that might arise. They later told me it was quite a battle to get Mom underground. Fortunately, since I was not there, it was easier for me.

The memorial service went smoothly. Vic did not attend. And since I skipped the graveside we both felt we had done our part.

Mom truly showed unconditional love. I never heard the term unconditional love come from her, but certainly saw her practice it. While I did not agree with everything she did or said, I had to admire her tireless efforts to help Vic.

In our society, we don't blame people if they can't run on broken legs, so why are we unable to understand that people can't make stellar decisions when they have broken minds?

Among the special people who tried to help my brother:

* Cecil Littlejohn, Vic's longtime employer, went so far as to pay Vic's child support so Vic wouldn't be in further trouble with the law. But, alas, when Vic found out what Cecil was doing he quit working for him.

* Cameron Littlejohn, Cecil's son, who let Vic live in his yard in a trailer.

* Harry Auble, who continues to give Vic a place in which to live and somehow manages to listen to his rants and raves.

I asked one of Harry's neighbors if he had ever heard Vic talk about diet. The neighbor chuckled and said he had heard Vic telling Harry, "If you want to live to be an old man, you have to eat right!" What made the scene funny was that Harry was already over 90 and probably didn't need any advice from Vic.

Chapter Seven

THE TARGETS

After Mom passed away, I was mad. The hard thing was figuring out whom to be most angry at.

Vic was sick and Mom had been trying to help Vic. So, in spite of the adverse effects their interactions had on our family, I could not justify feeling angry toward them.

How about Mom's landlords? What a perfect target they would be. That certainly would not include the apartment manager, Della. She truly had been an angel, looking after Mom and being a great help to us. In addition, all the tenants loved her.

The two men who purchased the apartment house in which Della worked were another matter. After Mr. Flintheart and Mr. Green (not their real names) closed the deal, they gave poor Della less than two weeks to move out and find a new job. Everyone was terribly sad about the way Della was being treated. Worse yet, the new landlords abused the tenants. Mom's neighbor told me they made a mockery of redecorating an apartment for an immigrant family by ripping wallpaper off one wall and applying it to another.

The landlords behaved strangely, relocating their office to the second floor and then displaying a shotgun outside the office. It was unclear how they expected people to have access to them, because the entrance to the building was by key only. And the shotgun was certainly intimidating.

Mom passed away on September 4, 1993 and had written her rent check for the full month of September. The neighbor had passed it on to the landlords. I was sure the landlords would refund much of the rent money when we vacated Mom's apartment. I told the neighbor to notify the landlords that we'd have Mom's apartment cleaned out by the middle of the month.

Imagine my surprise when the neighbor called to say that the landlords had packed Mom's belongings, told the tenants to take anything they wished and rented the apartment to a couple of drunks who annoyed the neighbors with their partying.

The tenants were sure the new owners were drug dealers and their suspicions seemed well founded. When I asked the tenants where the landlords were when Mom died, they responded, "They're up in the San Juan Islands involved in a drug deal."

What a mess! Realizing I had to take action before the end of the month, I called Mr. Flintheart and identified myself as the daughter of the late Mrs. Shumate. The minute he heard who I was, Flintheart affected a sympathetic voice and asked how I was. I replied that I was not very well at all, especially after hearing what he'd done with my mother's belongings.

I told him I expected to be reimbursed for half-a-month's rent, which was $162.50, plus the cleaning deposit of $200. To round things off, I added $12.50 for pain and suffering. The total came to $375.

Flintheart responded: "You have no right to call me up and demand money over the phone."

I replied: "You had no right to enter my mother's apartment, touch her things and offer to give them away."

He said: "You did not communicate with me."

I said: "You are not the kind of landlord who stands out in the front yard watering the flowers and is, therefore, easy to communicate with. I have been told you were up in the San Juan Islands working on a drug deal."

He said: "Are you calling me a drug dealer!"

I said: "No, but your tenants think you are."

He said: "I don't care what my tenants think."

I answered: "That's obvious. Otherwise you would conduct your business differently."

Flintheart hung up the phone on me,

I called back and said, "It's me again!"

Flintheart replied: "I guess we got cut off."

I said: "I want the money."

He said: "I can't communicate with you."

I said: "Just pay me."

He said: "We might get cut off again."

I said: "I'm thinking of suing you."

He said: "I'm going to have my lawyer call you."

I said: "Please do. I'm dying to talk to your lawyer."

He asked: "What's your name again?"

I said: "Alice Crooker."

He said: "A very appropriate name."

I said: "I look forward to hearing from your lawyer."

I gave him my work number and then called the police and said, "Please go down and get that weasel who owns the apartment house and throw him in jail." They asked me why they should do that and I said, "Because he took my deceased mother's things and said the neighbors could have whatever they wanted and then he rented out her apartment to someone else, despite the fact that she had paid for the entire month."

They said: "That's pretty cold! We'll get an officer to take your complaint."

I said: "You know what; I think I'll just wait. His stupid lawyer is going to call me and I will hear what he has to say first."

The police told me to call back if I needed them.

A man identifying himself as Flintheart's lawyer called me at work. I got right to the point. "Thank you for calling. Your client is stupid, craven and crass. And I will have you know that I will pursue him as long as I live because I am doing this in memory of my mother. I will never give up, so your client had better pay." Then I stopped for breath.

The man representing himself as "Mr. Flintheart's lawyer" replied, "I'm sure you will find my client is actually a wonderful person."

I wondered how, with Flintheart's track record, I was ever going to do that. So I told the man who called himself a lawyer that he should teach Mr. Flintheart the laws of the land when it came to business dealings. I added that if I were a greedy person I would allege that his client stole things that never even existed. For example, I could say, "Where are my mother's diamonds and fur coats?" While I would not do that, I added, I would alert the police. In fact, I already had. And furthermore, I was fully prepared to have his client jailed if he did not cooperate.

We agreed to meet at the apartment house at 4 p.m. Sunday. The man who said he was Mr. Flintheart's lawyer would, at that time, deliver my mother's things and hand me a check. I called Della and told her what had happened. She said, "Mr. Green's not a lawyer. He and Flintheart are roommates. When Flintheart is backed into a corner, he threatens people with Mr. Green." I was grateful for the information.

Dave and I talked over the situation. He was anxious to go with me to the Sunday meeting, armed with a shotgun. But since he was supposed to be at work on Sunday, I felt it best if he left his schedule intact. I also felt it would be much safer for all concerned if I got police protection. So I called and arranged to have an officer accompany me to my meeting with Mr. Green.

I arrived in town on Sunday and called for my escort. A policeman roughly the size of Godzilla met me in the Safeway parking lot. He also had a dog. I was thrilled. The only drawback, it turned out, was that the animal was not a trained "drug dog."

We entered the apartment house at the appointed hour and proceeded to the second floor, where we found a note on the door: "Working in the basement."

The officer said, "We'll go to the basement." We went into the basement, which was like a set from one of those old black-and-white mystery movies. The officer had his flashlight out, scanning the area as we walked.

When we failed to locate Mr. Green and Mr. Flintheart, I suggested that we ask Mom's neighbor if she knew where they were. When the neighbor opened the door and saw the policeman, she hugged me. I didn't want to disappoint her, but I told the neighbor that the policeman was protecting me and was not there to arrest either Green or Flintheart.

The policeman suggested we try the office again. We returned to the office and the policeman said, "Just open the door. After all, this is supposed to be an office."

The moment I opened the door, the grungy Mr. Green appeared. His face blanched pure white when he saw the policeman and I couldn't help feeling a little triumphant as I announced, "Don't worry. He's here to take care of me, not to arrest you." I paused and then added, "I couldn't trust you to do the right thing after you falsely represented yourself to me as a lawyer."

Green stammered, "Oh, I never said I was a lawyer."

I said, "Don't worry about it. I want the money and Mom's things."

Green got very busy writing the check and finding Mom's belongings. As he was doing this, the policeman looked around the place and evidently didn't like what he saw.

I had just finished saying to the policeman, "Just look at this mess. I sure wish your dog was a 'drug dog.'" At that moment the policeman pointed at a boot-covered foot protruding from behind the entrance to the next room and said, "I wonder what that is?"

I said, "Oh, it's probably Flintheart." I walked over and saw a man stretched out on a couch, his face covered with his hat. I said, "Good afternoon, Mr. Flintheart, Alice Crooker here. Sorry we couldn't meet under more pleasant circumstances."

Flintheart lifted his hat long enough to say, "I apologize."

I replied, "I will accept that."

While I went with Green to recover my mother's property, the policeman stayed behind to talk with Flintheart.

As we left, the policeman said, "I feel sorry for you."

I said, "All I want to do is get the stuff and get out of here."

As a result of my visit, the building inspector paid a visit to the apartment house and "failed" Flintheart and Green's so-called renovations. He also made the two men move their office back to the first floor.

I hope they learned to treat their tenants a little better.

In retrospect, the incident actually helped me through a difficult period. It gave me a focus for my anger. It also saved me from having to clean Mom's apartment.

Chapter Eight

THE CHARMED LIFE

By now, you are thinking, "What a life! Didn't anything good ever happen to this woman?" The answer is "Yes! I have lived a charmed life and have had more fun than almost anyone."

There is a reason I have had such a good life.

If you were to drop around our house in the evening, anytime after 7 p.m., you would quickly spot the cornerstone of my joy. If you have trouble seeing him, it is because he doesn't carry an extra ounce on his six-foot frame. Oh yes, and he's also handsome, blue-eyed and 25 percent hard-headed Norwegian. And I have adored David Crooker for the last 41 years.

Strangely enough, it was Vic who brought David into my life when I was about 16. For that, I am eternally grateful. Vic and Dave were friends, back when our families lived about 2 1/2 miles from each other in Washington State's Snoqualmie Valley. Both families attended the same church, and Vic and Dave hiked together and went target-shooting and generally had fun long before Vic's mental instability took over.

I was attracted to Dave from the start, but did my admiring from afar until he started coming to the house to see Vic. Sometimes Vic wasn't around. When that happened, Dave didn't immediately excuse himself by saying, "Guess I missed him, I'll be back later." Instead, he hung around to talk to me.

We found that we thoroughly enjoyed each other's company. Dave was a senior in the College of Forestry at the University of Washington and he spent a lot of time teaching me the botanical names of trees.

Dave's family knew how to live. They took family vacations. They went out to restaurants together. At Christmas they actually decorated their home and got dressed up and enjoyed themselves. This was a new concept for me, such a far cry from my own dysfunctional home that it seemed idyllic.

Nothing is perfect, I guess, because Dave's parents eventually divorced. But they were civilized about it and got on with their lives.

Mom was no help with my romance. In fact, it was surprising that Dave hung around. Mom was on a "Green Drink" kick when I first started going with Dave. And when Mom discovered a new "remedy," guaranteed to make one eternally healthy, she crusaded.

"Green Drink" was, indeed, something special! It consisted of ground comfrey mixed with pineapple juice. Mom offered it to Dave and he managed to choke it down. We later learned that the concoction is toxic to the liver.

Mom didn't succeed in killing Dave off and our love blossomed. On July 16, 1966, we were engaged to be married. Thirty-one days later, Uncle Sam snatched Dave, who had just earned his B.S. in Forestry. Vic had already been drafted and sent to Vietnam. I was terrified that Dave would soon be there.

After crying for days, I caught a glimpse of my sad face in the mirror. If I continued the way I was going, I would be so ugly by the time Dave returned that the last thing in the world he would want to do is marry somebody who looked like me.

Dave came home on leave from Fort Sam Houston, Texas where he had taken basic Army training while I worked halfheartedly on a B.S. degree in nursing. My mind was usually occupied with thoughts of marrying Dave and living happily ever after.

There was good news that fall. Dave had been accepted into an experimental program – known as Operation Whitecoat – at Fort Detrick in Frederick, Maryland. Furthermore, he would be staying there for the duration of his military obligation!

"Whitecoat" was a hush-hush operation, where only soldiers who were both non-smokers and lifetime non-drinkers of alcohol or caffeine would undergo tests to see how they reacted to minute amounts of biological agents used in warfare. As a Seventh-day Adventist and college graduate Dave, a pacifist, was suddenly in demand.

With Dave guaranteed to stay stateside, it seemed logical for us to end our agonizing separation and be married at Christmas.

I had planned a beautiful wedding, with trees as decorations and my attendants in red-velvet dresses. How clueless I was. How wrong I was.

My folks threw a fit when I notified them that Dave and I planned to marry during the Christmas season. Mom wrote me an extremely nasty letter in which she said that if we moved our wedding up to Christmas everyone would automatically think it was because I was pregnant.

Mom should have been a preacher. I have never heard a preacher explain anything half as well as she could. By the time she got through telling me HOW I was wrong, WHEN I was wrong, WHERE I was wrong and WHY I was wrong, I couldn't help but grasp the idea that she thought I was WRONG, and so it would always be whenever I did or even thought of doing anything that did not meet with her approval.

Mom's negative reaction shouldn't have come as a surprise. She'd been that way my entire life. But somehow I'd always managed to accept her disapproval a lot easier in the past. After all, any ordinary wimp – and I was certainly a wimp – can manage to eat an inordinate amount of peas for dinner or a full bowl of wheat germ for breakfast to make her mother happy, even if doing so is extremely distasteful. But allowing one's mother to dictate her marriage plans is quite another matter.

Dave was home for Christmas. And when he flew out on the last day of the year, we were unable to see each other again until he returned three days before our re-scheduled July 30 wedding. We were apart for seven months that seemed more like seven decades.

I dealt with the situation exactly as any other young woman in love would. I lived, breathed and ate only to stay alive so I could read letters from Dave. When one arrived, I would read it, then stash it under my pillow and sleep on it until the next one arrived. I would read the new letter and then remove the old letter from under my pillow, putting it in a safe place. The new letter would take its place under my pillow. Fortunately, Dave was a faithful letter writer.

It was a miracle Dave made it home in time for the wedding. He was flying military standby and when the plane landed in Chicago the passengers began to shift. Dave did not budge from his seat. He was wearing the mandatory full-dress uniform and knew that the minute every seat was filled, if just one more person entered the cabin, he would be forced to get off.

Dave had almost given up hope, as passengers continued to stream into the plane. But then the crowd thinned out and when he glanced around the cabin he could see that every seat was taken. He had an overwhelming feeling of relief when the plane backed away from the gate.

Our wedding weekend was frenzied. Mom and Dad had a transportation emergency when an axle and wheel broke off their car.

But when the wedding day arrived, there we all were in the tiny Snoqualmie Seventh-day Adventist Church. The place was packed with friends and well-wishers and Pastor Clyde Pray was on hand to marry us. Dave and I are both tall, and Pastor Pray is quite short. But he managed to carry it off very well, jumping up on a chair at the end of the service to give me a kiss.

We honeymooned for three days at Birch Bay, up near the Canadian Border. After returning to visit our folks for one night, we headed back to Dave's military base in Maryland. This time I didn't have to watch a plane take Dave away from me. This time I was able to board the plane with the man I loved and fly far, far away.

When we landed in Baltimore, I thought surely we must be in the middle of Africa, because it was so hot and muggy. While Dave tried to devise a plan for us to get from the airport to our apartment in Frederick, I sat with our luggage and answered questions.

In wartime people open up and bare their souls to strangers. One young soldier (they were all young) asked if I had recently gotten married. When I answered, "Yes," he asked how long we'd been married. When I told him, "Just three days," he asked if I liked being married. I told him it was "wonderful," and he relaxed sufficiently to tell me that he, too, was thinking of getting married.

Dave was getting a run-around concerning transportation. It still bothers us that because Dave was wearing a military uniform and his rank wasn't high enough, the car-rental people refused to rent him a car.

ALICE CROOKER

We kept looking longingly at the city buses as they pulled in and out. It was easy to see that the buses lacked sufficient room to accommodate us and all our possessions, so we had to forgo the most economical and convenient option.

In the midst of our dismay, the sky suddenly opened up and unleashed oceans of water. Thunder rolled. Lightning flashed. This did nothing to clarify our problem, which was simply how best to get from the airport to our apartment 40 miles away.

As if that weren't enough to worry about, the lightning reminded me of the untimely demise of Dave's great-grandmother on his mother's side. Dave's grandmother was only 12 years old when lightning hit his great-grandmother's home in Minnesota. The lightning knocked her unconscious and, despite the best efforts of man and medicine, she died.

I would think of her often when we were in the midst of still another thunderstorm in Frederick.

On this day, however, we wound up taking a limousine to the Greyhound Bus Depot. The limo driver was miffed that we didn't leave him a larger tip. We weren't being cheap; we simply didn't have much money.

We boarded the bus and finally arrived in Frederick, where we took a taxi to Stewart Manor, Apt. #49.

Dave needed to check in with the base, and since we had no car or telephone, we took off on foot to a shopping mall that had a pay phone. Between us and the shopping mall was a construction area that had a high mound of dirt. Finding no way around it, we set out to cross it, almost immediately sinking to our knees in mud.

I loved the apartment. Dave had picked it out and paid an extra month's rent so we could move right in. It was perfect in every way except for the rug on the living room floor. It was a ghastly yellow, had a long tear in it and was covered with grime.

We eventually purchased a neutral rug and stored the yellow one. I spent many hours hand-sewing window curtains.

For the first few weeks, we walked to stores and walked home again with all our purchases, including groceries. Just once we called a cab, because another thunder-and-lightning storm came up while we were carrying a load of food.

We ran short of cash while waiting for our money to be transferred between interstate banks. Things took a lot longer in those days, before computers came into our lives. We were so broke we decided to look through our wedding cards once more, just in case one or two might contain money we had overlooked. We found $50, which was like manna from heaven. Fifty dollars may not seem like much these days, but back then it bought well over a month's worth of groceries.

A kindly woman who worked in the lab with Dave took pity on me and sold us a Ford Falcon for $65. We were set. Our life of "travel" was about to begin.

We began by seeing the sights around Frederick. It wasn't far to Harper's Ferry and we loved to go there and walk across the train trestle and lounge around where the Potomac and Shenandoah Rivers merge. We went to Gettysburg, too, and became thoroughly immersed in Civil War history.

Not too far from Frederick was a wild-animal farm that boasted a King Cobra presentation. I still remember it in vivid detail. A cage containing the cobra was brought out and opened. Since the 17-foot snake did not immediately come forth, the snake handler reached in with a stick and poked around. This stirred the snake to action and we saw him lunge forward, out of the cage and land with a thud on the green grass. The brave snake handler caught the snake by the back of the neck with his bare hands and put a glass jar to its mouth. The snake bit down on a piece of rubber that stretched across the top of the jar and released drops of venom into the jar – a procedure known as "milking the snake."

We were curious to learn how the man could turn loose of the snake without being bitten. It was quite simple really. A huge garbage can was brought in and the snake handler put the snake into it, tail first, and then wound the snake's massive body around and around in the garbage can. At the last moment, the snake handler threw the snake's head over and down. An attendant then quickly slammed the lid down on the snake and everyone breathed a sigh of relief.

Many years later, we returned to Maryland to show our two children the sights. We hoped to show them the King Cobra presentation, but found that the snake show had been discontinued. A woman told us the snake had grown to 20 feet and been taken to a zoo, because people no longer had any interest in seeing people handle large snakes.

Frederick was a fun place for newlyweds. The people at the Seventh-day Adventist Church took us under their wing and provided us with many delicious meals and hours of entertainment.

We went sightseeing as often as possible and on a visit to the Washington D.C. Zoo even managed a quick look at Smokey the Bear, who by this time was a very old, tired mascot.

We loved Washington D.C. and spent weekends visiting the museums, monuments and government buildings. On one visit to the U.S. Senate, we were sitting in the visitors' balcony watching the proceedings on the floor. We were informed that an important message was coming from then President Johnson. A page strode in, bowed and grandly stated, "A message from the President." As we puffed up thinking that it was something about Viet Nam and how we would hear it first hand, we were told our time was up. We had to leave.

Oh well, the cherry blossoms were beautiful and we could admire them endlessly. We climbed the Washington Monument and went through the White House. Unfortunately, Resurrection City went in and our tourism of D.C. ground down—too dangerous

The year we spent in Frederick flew by. Soon it was time for Dave to be discharged from the service. We decided to return home by driving through every New England state, crossing into Canada and then heading west until we reached Washington State. The Falcon was deemed too unreliable and underpowered to make the long trip west. We had traded for a 1965 Rambler Classic, practically a new car, and we were feeling quite uppity.

The travel itinerary went well for almost one full day. The muffler forgot its function and began to rumble. Two days later the muffler quit rumbling and started roaring. In Biddeford, Maine, we bought a new muffler for $44. Plans immediately changed. No longer able to afford a leisurely sightseeing journey home, we settled on a more direct route – straight up to Canada and then due west. We spent a delightful night in a lodge in Sturgeon Falls, Ontario, where the fire escape consisted of a rope hanging from a window.

I began the next morning by locking myself in the restroom of a Sturgeon Falls gas station. Dave to the rescue! There was a lot of rain that day and the road washed out about 60 miles east of Sault Ste. Marie, Ontario. There were no alternate routes, so we sat in the car for eight hours while road crews dumped rocks into the water. Truckers opened their trailers and tried to sell their wares. Bakery trucks sold Twinkies. Newspaper vendors went up and down the line selling to a captive audience.

While seated in the car we reached another decision. Canada was nice, but U.S. highways are not only infinitely better but far more plentiful. On the map it looked like a lot of miles of empty highway around the north side of Lake Superior. So, when the road re-opened we dipped down into Sault Ste. Marie, Michigan. There, for the second time in one day, I managed to lock myself in the women's restroom. This time the proprietors of the bed and breakfast helped Dave free me.

Both roads and car held up the rest of the way to Washington State, where it was time for Dave to begin job-hunting.

Chapter Nine

THE ACTIVE LIFE

Dave got a job as a forester with the Timber Department of Northern Pacific Railroad. This was the beginning of a long and satisfying career that spanned over thirty-six years with the same firm, now called Plum Creek Timber Company.

We settled in Buckley, Washington, a quiet little town in Pierce County with a gorgeous view of snow-capped Mt. Rainier, one of the truly majestic peaks in the Cascade mountain range, which stretches from Canada to Northern California. Mt. Rainier rises 14,411 feet above sea-level and is home to 26 officially named glaciers and numerous unnamed permanent ice fields. The mountain is massive with over 35 square miles of ice (The Challenge of Rainier by Dee Molenaar). Both Buckley and neighboring Enumclaw are built on the Osceola mud flow, a deposit from a long-ago cataclysmic eruption of what we native Puget Sounders call simply "The Mountain."

No other words are necessary. "The Mountain" is our Everest. It dominates the landscape in Buckley and nearly every home has a view. Mt. Rainier National Park, one of the oldest in the national park system, is also a wonderful place to visit. We often took day-hikes around Carbon Glacier and Mowich Lake.

One memorable weekend, after deciding we needed to test ourselves with something more than just a day-hike, we loaded up our backpacks and headed up to beautiful Spray Park, about four miles from the Mowich Lake parking lot. The weather was lovely and the view spectacular. We saw some signs of bears and decided against taking food into our homemade tent.

We were peacefully asleep under the stars that night when we were suddenly awakened by a crash that sounded like a falling tree. The tent moved and shook. Dave thought I was trying to get outside. But it wasn't me making the noise. We had a visitor. A bear!

I immediately thought of the orange peelings in my coat pocket and hoped they were not high on a bear's list of favorite foods.

I whispered to Dave that it was a time to pray and he whispered to me, "Don't you dare scream." There was a brief respite when the bear took Dave's backpack off into the woods. But it was short-lived. The bear returned after eating almost everything inside the backpack. Surely there must be more food somewhere! He lumbered around the tent, sniffing noisily. I continued to pray!

Finally the bear tired of the game and went away. I told Dave, "I'm going to the car."

Dave replied, "You'll run into the bear on the trail before you get to the car."

I know what it is to pray without ceasing, because I prayed the rest of the night. The Good Lord, knowing I could not have endured another visit from the bear, heeded my prayers.

We learned in the morning that the bear had visited our campground neighbors, who had a fire going. Because of the fire, they felt less threatened by the bear. We also discovered that the bear had dragged Dave's backpack about 300 feet from our tent, wrecking the pack's zipper and devouring most of its contents. The bear's powerful jaws had chewed right through a can of baked beans. The only thing unscathed was a little plastic bear filled with honey. I laughed and said the bear showed respect for its own kind.

We had nothing with which to make breakfast, so it was a long hike to our car. On the way, I warned everyone who passed us to be careful, because there was a bear up there somewhere! Dave told me to stop being a party pooper, but I wished someone had warned us ahead of time.

When we got home, we read in the newspaper that in another area of the national park a bear was inspecting a picnic table when a camper looked out of his tent to see what was happening. The bear lumbered over to the man and slapped him across the face. It took more than 20 stitches to close the claw marks.

We learned that if a bear becomes a nuisance, park officials will move it to the back country. Bears that are not afraid of people are very dangerous. We decided after our bear experience that we would do no more back country camping in national parks.

Even though we no longer felt the urge to camp in the park, we were still fascinated by The Mountain's snow and rock and crevasses. There was only one thing to do: Climb it! All 14,411 feet of it, if possible.

As the largest glaciated peak in the continental U.S., Mt. Rainier's summit is a worthy goal of both the highly skilled and the amateur climber. Despite its majestic beauty, it claims the lives of several climbers each year – both experienced and inexperienced.

The two main high camps are Muir and Schurman. The most frequently traveled route to the summit goes through Camp

Muir, on the south side of the mountain. One day, Dave and I hiked up to Muir, above the 10,000-foot mark, to see what it felt like at that altitude. Being at the camp also afforded us an opportunity to see guided climbing parties on their way down the mountain. From what we could see, the guides acted surly and superior toward the climbers. We decided that there was no way we would have guides take us to the summit. We would do it on our own when the time came.

We had it all planned out. During one of our vacations, we'd climb Glacier Peak, another of Washington State's 10,000-foot-plus volcanoes. That would give us the experience to tackle Rainier.

To prepare for Glacier Peak, we began running. I felt funny during a run one day and decided to check with a doctor. I was pregnant. The doctor said, "Whatever you do, don't climb any mountains now. I'm worried about a first-trimester miscarriage."

Although surprised, I was thrilled to be pregnant. Almost immediately complications set in and I spent most of that summer in bed. By September, we found that the pregnancy was over. There would be no baby. The doctor told me to resume my normal activities and try again for a baby.

In 1971, a beautiful, red-haired girl was born to Dave and me. We named her Becky and she was the pride and joy of our life. We were living in one of the oldest houses in Buckley at the time, and it was definitely not child-friendly. We found a builder and he constructed us a lovely little rambler with a view of Mt. Rainier.

We were scheduled to move into our "mansion" when an old friend, Ward Wilson, the father of my college roommate, called and invited us to join him on a climb of Mt. Rainier. He was the reluctant leader of a bunch of novices and wanted some reliable climbers as well as companionship on the trip. He wanted Dave to help him with the climb and agreed to take me on as well.

We jumped at the opportunity, even though it came at a bad time. There was the matter of moving into our new house the weekend before the climb. But, hey, we were young and invincible – we thought.

The difficulty of moving from one dwelling to another seems to be inversely related to the distance between the two houses. I have noticed that if one is only going around the corner, there seems to be no reason to pack carefully and efficiently.

Thus, we wound up taking far more trips and spending far more time than was necessary. In addition, Dave was in the midst of building a masterpiece of a canoe out of ¾-inch-wide strips of redwood. We couldn't just move this any old way. So, after easing the canoe onto the back of a pickup, I held one end of it and walked behind the truck to the new house.

We had purchased a freezer, paid to have it delivered to our old house and purposely left it crated so we would be certain to get it to our new house undamaged. After we loaded it on the truck, hauled it around to the new house and unloaded it, we discovered a huge dent in the side.

I called the vendor to complain and he said, "We'll send someone out to assess the damage and give you a partial refund."

I replied, "I don't want a dented freezer."

And he said, "O.K. Bring it back and we'll give you a new one."

I said, "You need to come and get it, because I paid to have it delivered."

The vendor replied, "We don't do things that way!"

We ended up having to haul the dented freezer back to the store. We then had to haul the new one back to our new house. Oh, the joy of loading and unloading! To top it off, I managed to come down with a nasty head cold. On the bright side, our dream of climbing to the top of Mt. Rainier was almost within our grasp.

The ascent was to be from the Camp Schurman side of the mountain, a route that is longer than approaching from Camp Muir but technically less difficult.

Getting up to Camp Schurman at 9,500 feet was a cakewalk for me. Part of the fun was crossing the crevasses, which can be tricky. They are usually hidden by snow, and as the day wears on and the snow softens they can be treacherous.

Our experienced climbers would usually approach a crevasse, scratch their heads and ponder the best way to cross it. By the time I got to the crevasse and yelled, "What shall I do?"

They would reply, "Just step across it, Alice."

I was traveling along, smugly wondering why it was so difficult for them to cross the crevasses and so easy for me to do it, when the rope suddenly went tight. I stopped and looked at the climber behind me to see what his problem was. I could see him only from the waist up.

"I'm in a crevasse," he said. I started to yell. Once again the experienced climbers laughed and said, "Just step across it, Alice."

I yelled back. "There is nothing to step across. Come and get this guy out of the hole he's fallen into, for Pete's sake."

It wasn't long before Ward, our climb leader, stepped into a crevasse. Fortunately, only one leg went in – up to the hip.

We reached Camp Schurman and ate supper. The summit ascent was to begin at 1 o'clock the next morning. We bedded down about 7 p.m. and tried to sleep, our minds racing with thoughts of what awaited us the next day. Dave and I were on the top floor of a two-story hut and our sleep was disrupted by some late-arriving climbers, who began cooking and talking. The bacon they were frying was especially unappealing to me.

Too soon, it was time to arise and ascend. I arose, but the ascension was where the trouble began. A gentleman on my rope team was petrified that I would not be able to stop him if he fell. He kept trying to impress on me how to hold the rope and eyed me with great trepidation. I did not want him to be nervous. So, to demonstrate my climbing proficiency and etiquette I put my flashlight (we did not have headlamps in those days) down beside the next crevasse so he could see that nothing stood between me and his safety.

I was horrified when I saw my flashlight roll over and slide down the crevasse. This unnerved me. I was now climbing with less than optimum light and feeling freaky. One of the rope teams moved in beside me so I could benefit from its light.

After a few hours I was exhausted. My feet were stepping up and plunking down in the same spot. Ward towed me for a while, until his knees gave out.

We stopped to rest on Emmons Glacier at approximately 12,500 feet. One of the climbers poked his ice axe into the snow while he rested. The axe kept going down, into a hidden crevasse. At that point, our party decided to turn back. Some of the climbers were not happy with the decision, but under the circumstances it seemed the wisest thing to do.

As I looked around and down – and there was a lot of "down" to see – I felt like a cat up a tree, with no way to get down. I looked at Dave and started to cry. I whimpered, "I want to see Becky again!"

Dave had the perfect comeback. He looked around calmly and said, "I think this is about where they found Delmar Fadden frozen in the snow." In 1936, poor Delmar Fadden had attempted a solo winter ascent of Mt. Rainier without first notifying the Park Service of his intentions. He had attained the summit and was descending when he apparently lost a crampon and fell. His body was spotted from a plane five days later and subsequently recovered by a rescue team .

I snapped, "You shut-up, Dave. I'm going to get down!" Then I looked at Ward and said, "Don't go too fast, I don't want to fall."

We began a nightmarish descent. Ward had taken codeine for the pain in his knees and it supercharged him. Whenever he approached a crevasse, he jumped like he was attempting to leap across the Grand Canyon. When I saw him jump like that, I abandoned all hope of making it. But when I got there, I would discover that all I needed to do was "step across it, Alice!"

We finally made it back to Camp Schurman, where we rested and packed the remainder of our gear. We were fed up with crevasses and decided to climb up and over a prominent rock called Steamboat Prow. We could not have made a worse choice. The climb was difficult and the terrain unsafe. Parts of the route had us walking on crumbly, shifting rock.

I had rented boots from REI (Recreational Equipment, Inc.) and by that time my feet were killing me. The moment I got below the snow, off came the boots and I walked barefoot for two miles.

As we slowly descended, I vowed to stay away from the summit of Mt. Rainier – forever. I would enjoy it from afar. I have managed to honor my vow except for a recurring dream in which I climb toward the summit with ease. But for some reason I always wake up before I reach the summit.

Even though I didn't make it to the top of Rainier, I was pleased with the effort I put forth. And I'm always quick to let people know that once, long ago, I came close.

Chapter Ten

THE BEST OF TIMES

Contrary to the opinion of my eighth grade teacher, the best thing I ever did was to become pregnant. I looked and felt the best of my entire life, and would gladly do it all again. The best times were with the children. As I mentioned, we had Becky in 1971. Along came Dan in 1975. I was very fortunate to be a stay-at-home Mom and the kids and I had oodles of fun.

I could never understand my teacher who lacked in about every way imaginable. She seemed to get her kicks out of life by putting down or hitting kids. In my minds eye, I can almost hear the board interview she underwent to get the job. "Do you hate and oppose children?"

"Yes, to the utmost, in every way, every second of every minute of every day. Even on the weekends, I catch myself plotting against the little devils!"

"Good, you are hired! Keep on with your opposition and all should go very well."

All went, but, I can't say well. If we had only been old people instead of children, there would have been no problem at all.

It seemed as though we never really did anything except prepare to live and I used to wonder when we could begin to live.

We were supposed to make a scrapbook and I made a beautiful one. It had a picture of a healthy looking "spinach man," on the front cover. In case one is unfamiliar with a spinach man, it was only a cartoon man growing out of a spinach leaf. Since the subject was health, leave it to me to have a real picture of health. I wood-burned the picture and was excited, happy, and yes, even proud, of my book.

The next assignment was to put in the book a picture of what we wished to be when we grew up. I thought this was so easy; the good old Sears catalogue had the perfect photo. I had only one goal in life and that was to have children, so I opened the catalogue, turned quickly to the maternity clothes section and spied a happy-looking pregnant woman, cut her out and glued her in.

I thought the teacher would love my book, I thought wrong!

She flared her nostrils at me and spoke with great disdain. "Why did you put that awful picture in there? What were you thinking of? These books will be on display at Camp Meeting!" Camp Meeting was our church's annual state wide gathering of up to 3000 members. "What will all the people think when they see this book? What will they think of you, the school, me as a teacher?"

I visualized a long line of mad people and changed the picture. I wish I had stuck to my guns, because it was what I wanted and I am glad I accomplished it. There! It didn't make the scrapbook, but – in concept at least – it made this book.

I liked to go with the kids on their outings, and every year I accompanied them to the Puyallup Fair, Western Washington's major fall extravaganza. I also was the school's fund-raiser and eventually chaired the school board for a year. Dave and I also worked with the kids at church, playing games and telling stories.

Not only did we have bountiful Christmases, but when we moved into our present house in Kirkland, with its high-vaulted ceiling, we were able to have a 14-foot tree. It usually took me several days of climbing up and down a ladder to do the decorating.

Dave also saw to it that we took regular family vacations. For years we went, without fail, to Lincoln City on the Oregon Coast. There, we walked the beach, flew kites and waded in the cold Pacific Ocean. We took the children with us to Hawaii, which provided us with a family joke that still makes us laugh. Five-year-old Dan, in all seriousness, said to Becky, "Let's pretend we're swimming in Hawaii."

We camped in the outdoors and made speeches around the campfire at night. The speech game was our own invention. We'd assign a topic to the family member whose turn it was; give him or her a few minutes to think and then sit back to listen to an impromptu speech – often with hilarious results.

It was at Expo '86 in Vancouver, B.C. that the entire family – with the exception of me – turned into devotees of that fair's Scream Machine, a wild, looping roller coaster. Becky was the first to try it, when I drove her and some school friends to the fair for an eighth-grade graduation party. When we later made the trip as a family, Becky talked so much about the Scream Machine that her brother said he'd take the ride with her.

However, when we arrived at the fair, Dan took one look at the Scream Machine and decided it was not for him. Since I had already assured Becky there was no way I would go with her, that left Becky's father.

Dave looked the ride over and agreed to accompany his daughter. He found it to be so much fun, in fact, that he and Becky taunted Dan into trying it. Nervous at the outset, Dan soon got into the spirit of the ride and he was jubilant when the ride came to an end.

Now they all started in on me. Was I going to be the family party-pooper? I hated to be the only one not to try it, so I climbed aboard reluctantly. While the rest of the family whooped and hollered, I sat mute. When the coaster dropped down while careening around a corner, Dave expected noise from me. Hearing nothing, he yelled, "Are you there?"

I replied, "Where else would I be. It's not like I can say, I've had enough. Thank you very much; I will get off here NOW! I REALLY MEAN NOW WHEN I SHOUT NOW!!"

Dave said, "Hang on, here comes the good part." The "good part" was the gravity-defying-loop part of the ride. I was immensely relieved to get off that ride and back on solid ground.

We also went to Disneyland as a family and quickly became addicted. Our home is frequently referred to as the Mickey Mouse house because of all the Disney-inspired decorations I have put up.

In 1993, we sent Becky for one quarter of her junior year to Newbold College in Bracknell, Berkshire, England. I went over to visit her for Mother's Day and thus began my love affair with this charming country. May, in England, is beautiful. The rhodies were in full bloom, the fields all yellow with something exotic. I rented a car and drove Becky and her roommate nearly 1200 miles in the little time I was there. We went to Land's End and even took a boat out to the Scilly Isles.

Dave and I sat down one day to set some travel goals. High on our list was Tahiti and the nearby islands in French Polynesia. We had read *The Bounty Trilogy* and wondered what it would be like to see the area first-hand.

Our dream came true in 1994. Becky was graduating from college and Dan from high school, and we finally had an excuse for our family's dream trip. After many hours on Air France, where we watched an arrow move far too slowly down the map along the Chilean Coast and finally across the Pacifc, we landed in Papeete, Tahiti. We climbed aboard a small commuter plane and finally, after a brief stop on another island, landed on a World War II landing strip on one of the motus surrounding the volcanic island of Bora Bora. We were then transported by launch to exotic Hotel Bora Bora.

We spent several nights at the Hotel Bora Bora, purportedly where the rich and famous stay. Although we were neither rich nor famous, we were treated royally.

Bora Bora is northwest of Tahiti in the Society Islands. When we arrived at our hotel, we were informed that our garden bungalows were unavailable. Not to worry. We would be put up instead in over-the-water bungalows for most of our stay – at no extra charge. We were thus able to snorkel right off our own dock into a coral garden. Fresh flowers and fruits were placed in the room daily. It was unbelievable.

One day we were taken out in the lagoon, where a rope was stretched out in front of us. We donned our snorkeling gear and held onto the rope while sharks were fed on the other side. I guess the sharks knew not to cross under the rope!

Bora Bora is about 17 miles in circumference and we wanted to explore the entire island. Ignoring warnings about the tiny mopeds (motorized scooters) used by the natives, we decided to rent them. We were mature, responsible people, what could happen? Since there were only two mopeds available, it was agreed that Dave and I would make the first trip around the island. The kids could do it after we finished.

Being nervous, I drove so slowly at the outset that the moped almost tipped over. Dave said, "Speed up, Alice." So I increased my speed and soon had the hang of staying upright. We made it almost all the way around the island before stopping for a snack, at which time I said boastfully, "I am so proud of myself. I can ride a moped and some people, I understand, have awful wrecks."

That, of course was the wrong thing to say. In trying to get up a small embankment to the road from the gravel parking lot where we had stopped to eat, I gave the moped a little too much gas. Bam! I was down in the middle of the street.

Dave had heard the crash and turned around to see a cop looking at me. My pants had a hole ripped in them, my knee was bloody and the moped definitely needed help. This must have been a common occurrence since the cop neither offered to help or reprimand me.

Pride does, indeed, go before a fall.

Chapter Eleven

SPREADING THE DOOM

I was cloaked in a pall of gloom and doom as I pulled into the driveway of our home. A diagnosis of Parkinson's does that to you. The future was uncertain and the unknown is always frightening.

It occurred to me that I needed to let Dave know what was going on. I rang his office, only to discover that he had been through an ordeal of his own that morning.

A group of activists concerned about the impact of tree-cutting on the area's wildlife had descended on company headquarters to air their concerns. The police had arrived to keep order and Dave was in the lobby answering questions and explaining the timber industry's position.

One questioner asked Dave if logging decisions, some of which could lead to the demise of woodland creatures, weren't comparable to a parent deciding which of his children would be saved in a disaster. "Did he think he was God?"

When Dave picked up the phone to answer my call, he had forgotten I was to see the doctor that day. He was more stunned than I had been over the lousy news.

That evening we went to a bookstore and bought a copy of Glenna Wotton Atwood's wonderful book, *Living Well With Parkinson's*. This book has been a great help to me. The courageous author encourages those with Parkinson's to be open about their condition. We took her advice.

The people where I worked knew, of course, that something was wrong with me and it most likely was something major. But there were others to think of too. I was committed to help with a bridal shower at church and also scheduled for an MRI on the same day. Obviously some things would have to be cut from my schedule. The most reasonable explanation would be to tell people the truth.

We have no regrets about stating the facts early on, because Parkinson's victims are better able to deal with the reactions of others before they become noticeably impaired.

Still, I was so angry with the diagnosis that I was filled with rage. Looking back, I can see how shocked people were when I said, "Guess what! I might have Parkinson's disease or a brain tumor! By the way, I hope it's a brain tumor, because I know of people who have had brain tumors fixed."

Many of my friends, relatives and associates may very well have had serious problems of their own to deal with and I wasn't handling mine very well.

While I didn't want anyone to self-destruct over my diagnosis, I also didn't want people to airily dismiss it as "no problem" or to say, "Just be glad it isn't something worse."

Still grasping at straws, I tried to convince myself that the doctor had become bored with diagnosing "simple" neurological disorders and had decided to add some spice to his life by saying I had "Parkinson's." Sure, that was probably it. I could hardly wait for my insurance company to set him straight. Parkinson's indeed! All the MRI's and lab tests required for a suspected case of Parkinson's would cost a bundle.

Alas, my insurance company failed me. A receptionist called to say the company had been unable to talk with my doctor. The doctor's receptionist, on the other hand, assured me that the doctor had, indeed, talked with the insurance company and received approval to proceed with all the needed procedures.

This battle went on for some time – the doctor's office saying the procedures had been approved, the insurance company's spokesperson saying they had not. The problem had to be cleared up soon because I was scheduled for an MRI.

Several days before the MRI was due, the receptionist from the imaging firm called to say my insurance company still hadn't given its approval. "Good," I said. "I don't want to have it anyway. Just cancel it."

The caller laughed nervously and said, "Why don't you check it out with your insurance company." So I called the insurance company and was told, "No problem. Your procedure has been approved." I asked the insurance company if they would be so kind as to call the lab and relay the news and was told, "No, it's your job to call the lab and relay that information."

So, I called the lab and relayed the information. That wasn't sufficient, I was told. A representative of the insurance company had to personally call and guarantee payment.

The day before I was to report for the scan, the receptionist at the imaging firm called and said, "Don't bother to come. Your insurance company still hasn't approved the procedure."

I replied, "I'm coming anyway. I know I'm covered. I've been assured they will pay. Furthermore, my husband has been given time off from work to accompany me.

The MRI was not my idea of fun, since I am severely claustrophobic and the only way I could tolerate 45 minutes inside that noisy machine was for Dave to stand nearby, reach into the machine and hold my hand. Today the MRI machines are much improved and they cause me no difficulty—they are roomy! I do not wish for anyone to fear an MRI. Be glad for the technology.

The results of the MRI were negative, which meant that despite my fervent wish there was no brain tumor. Everything was normal. It was becoming increasingly obvious that the doctor's preliminary diagnosis of Parkinson's disease was 100 percent correct.

When the doctor's receptionist called and asked me to repeat a blood test, because something in my liver looked fishy, I was overjoyed. "Hey," I said, still grasping at straws, "Maybe I have Wilson's disease."

The surprised receptionist said, "Why do you want to have a disease?"

I replied, "Because I have a disease that I don't like and would prefer something else."

With that the receptionist glanced at my chart and said, "Oh, I see that you have Parkinson's."

I paid a return visit to my doctor, who told me that an irregularity in my lab tests had set him to wondering if I might possibly have lupus. He'd sent my lab work to the University of Washington and had been informed that there was no sign of lupus.

With that the doctor sat back, very composed, and listened to me vent. My last hope seemed to be gone. Nevertheless, I wouldn't give up without a fight. "Parkinson's is such a stupid disease," I said. "Can't you think of anything better than Parkinson's?"

"No," he said, "I cannot." Then he asked me what I would prefer it to be.

I realized he'd put me on the spot intentionally. But I fooled him by asking him the one question that most doctors hate to hear.

"Have you ever made a mistake and misdiagnosed anyone?"

He replied, "Of course I have. I am not God." He then encouraged me to seek a second opinion.

I was impressed with his honesty and realized it was not his fault I had Parkinson's disease. Since I saw no reason to "shoot the messenger," I stayed with him.

About two years after the MRI, I arrived home from work with thoughts of a pleasant, relaxing evening. Dave, who had arrived home a short time earlier, said, "Do you know a Mr. Burns? He left you a menacing phone message!"

I listened to the message and agreed with Dave. Mr. Burns did not sound happy. I returned his call straightaway.

It turned out that Mr. Burns was a collection agent – a very heavy handed one. He informed me that I owed $900 dollars and some odd change. Furthermore, the entire sum was due and payable that very day. No matter that it was now after 7:00 p.m.

When I asked "to whom do I owe this money?" he snarled, "You had an MRI."

I said, "Oh, do they do their billing through a collection agency?"

He replied, "They couldn't find you."

I said, "My insurance company took care of this a long time ago. I will call the MRI people tomorrow. I will not deal with a collection agency because I have perfect credit."

The collection agent retorted, "Not after today, you won't."

"Fine," I replied and hung up the phone.

The moment I arrived at work the next morning, I told my co-workers about Mr. Burns' threat. Then I called the billing department for the imaging lab and asked what in the world was going on and why was I being accosted by a collection agent.

They were able to tell me that they had transposed the numbers of our mailing address and had received mail back for two years. I asked why they hadn't bothered to consult a telephone directory to check out our address and was told, "We don't have time to do such things."

When I asked what I should do to straighten out the problem, I was told to pay the collection agency. I responded that there was no way I would do such a thing. Then I was told that I could just pay the lab directly if the collection agent bothered me.

I told them I had a better idea. I was going to hire a lawyer.

The person handling my call issued a challenge of her own, "Go right ahead then."

After that unsatisfactory verbal exchange, I rang the MRI lab again and asked for the manager of collections. When she came on the line, I took a different approach. Why on earth had I been accosted by a thug over a bill that I was unaware of? Why was I threatened with ruination of my heretofore spotless credit rating? And why should I, a reasonable person, think I owed them anything? After all, I had received their original bill and had also received notice that the insurance company had paid 80 percent of the charge. When I heard nothing further, I presumed that the MRI lab was fully satisfied with the payoff. Could I please have an itemized bill and be removed from the clutches of the collection agent?

The manager of collections was apologetic and quickly agreed to remove me from any more contact with the collection agency. She did not know how she could furnish me with an itemized bill and was surprised when I told her that if she could tell me what the insurance company had paid, I could quickly tell her what my 20 percent payment should be. I added that I

PEAS, "PILLS," AND PARKINSON'S

would like to take up the matter of timeliness. Just how long should a person have to wait to receive a bill? And why did a person have to be treated so rudely?

While I was on the phone with the MRI lab, who should call the store where I worked and begin to grill amiable salesperson Rick about Alice Crooker? Why, it was none other than the churlish Mr. Burns. Did a person named Alice Crooker work there? And if so, how much money did she make?

Rick was perfect. He replied that I worked there, but he was clueless as to how much I made because I was the accountant and wrote all the paychecks. Poor Mr. Burns hung up with a "harrumph!"

I rang the collection agency and said, "You can tell your weasel, Mr. Burns, to please get his nose out of my business and quit harassing me. Also, you can remove me from your collection list, because I am working directly with the MRI lab to resolve the mix-up."

The receptionist replied that my name would be removed from the list when "we feel like it."

The whole injustice of the situation weighed heavily on me. I, of course, expressed my displeasure everywhere I went. My friends did not hold out much hope for me getting away without paying, but I said, "We'll just wait and see."

At such times I turn the impossible over to God. It is not bribing Him; it is just a partnership with Him. I say, "All right, God, here's the deal. I would much rather give you the money than these people. So, if you fix it so I don't have to pay, I will give you $100."

I don't worry about the situation and it has never failed to turn out for the best. In this case, I ended up paying the MRI service $26.50. That left me $73.50 for God. I was so happy.

It's been said that man's extremity is God's opportunity, and I need to make very clear that if it were not for the grace of God, I would have given up a long time ago.

Since God is in charge, I always have hope.

Chapter Twelve

COULD BE WORSE

When I was diagnosed with Parkinson's disease, I wish I could say I rose heroically to the occasion. I wish I had reacted with grace and dignity by saying something like: "Whew, I'm so glad it isn't worse," or "I'm so fortunate; there are so many people much worse off than I." But, since this is non-fiction, I will have to stick with the facts.

In truth, my reaction could not have been worse. I am at a loss tó explain my frustration. The English language does not contain sufficient nuances for me to adequately describe my fear and dismay.

While I walked around smiling, pretending I had the best attitude imaginable, I was inwardly obsessed with death. How could I die?

Poor Dave bore the brunt of it all and I don't know how he stood it. One day, as we were riding in the car, I looked over at Dave and said, "I know what to do. When I get bad with this disease, I will attack you and say I am about to kill you. Then you can kill me and get off on self-defense." Dave did not appreciate my suggestion.

I could not kill myself because suicide is contrary to my personal convictions. I believe God should determine the length of my life. But just because I do not believe in suicide does not mean the idea did not enter my head. My imagination is always active. Thank goodness I do not follow through on everything that pops into my mind. Actually, what I was doing was looking into the future, realizing I would someday become a heavy burden on my family and friends and wanting to spare them the trouble.

Because of my growing-up years, in which my parents stressed that only work has value, I could not conceive of any role in society other than "working like a dog."

I had studied at the feet of a master, my mother, who did not content herself with simply vacuuming, dusting and picking up clutter in a reasonable manner. Mom attacked those tasks with demonic intent, overdoing them as she did everything else in life. She scrubbed every inch of our ceilings and walls because our wood stove smoked things up. Before long, of course, ceilings and walls were dirty again. But, instead of replacing the stove, she re-tackled walls and ceilings as if driven by Simon Legree. It was, therefore, impossible for me to imagine a life that was not filled with frenzied activity.

The other problem was that if I ever became sick, it was my fault. My mother said so! If I had eaten better, slept better, or somehow or someway done things differently I would never get sick. My mother was convinced that a lack of Vitamin E had caused me to grow so tall (5'-10") and awkward, overlooking the simple genetic fact that my father was tall.

Genetics also played a role in the extreme height (6'-8") of Dave's and my son, Dan.

In our family, sudden death was not uncommon. Great Uncle Judge keeled over and died in a lawyer's office. Uncle Judge's brother, Clarence, fell into a fire while burning some trash. He died immediately. With those examples before me, the idea of becoming a long-term burden on my husband and children held no appeal.

On "Doomsday," when the dreaded diagnosis of Parkinson's disease was confirmed I reacted with tears. When the doctor said, "It could be worse," he was right. But it also could have been much better. I would like to erase from our vocabulary the words "could be worse," because to me they are cold and uncaring. If people wish to apply those words to their own condition, that's fine with me. I would much prefer to hear, "I am so sorry. I wish things could be better for you."

It did not take me long to find that things "could be worse." As chairperson of a church board, I became aware that instead of dealing with the reality of people in the congregation who were hurting, many of the "saints of the church" preferred to spend their time criticizing the preacher and complaining about petty issues.

One board member expressed concern about the church's shut-ins and wanted us to discuss ways to care for their needs. It sounded like a good idea to me, but the other board members showed absolutely no interest. When the issue came up at a subsequent meeting, and there was still no interest, I said, "Fine, I'll visit them myself."

My first visit was to a parishioner with end-stage Parkinson's. He had been very active in our church and a revered teacher. But I found him literally frozen in bed, his mouth stuck open. He was obviously miserable.

My second visit was to a certifiable genius, a retired physicist, who also had Parkinson's. He was able to talk well enough to let me know he was unable to swallow his own saliva and it took him 20 minutes to walk to the bathroom.

I was horror stricken after the visits, convinced I would wreck Dave's life. I called my primary-care physician and told him I could not go on living.

The doctor responded, "Alice, first you need to come to China with me and see how miserable the people are there before they die."

I replied, "At least they're on the right track. They're dying."

The doctor answered, "Your attitude is terrible. What would you do if you had some horrible cancer or heart trouble?"

I responded, "Then I would either get well or I would die and be done with it."

He said, "You are so morbid that you will wreck Dave's life and you will wreck it right now. Everyone will die sometime."

I shot back, "You are on the wrong train. I am not worried about dying. I am worried about living. I am afraid to live."

He said, "Well, today is all you have. Look at me. I will probably die of prostate cancer. Should I worry about that today?"

I said, "No, but I happen to be an accountant and I fix things. If something is wrong I find it and I fix it and I like everything to add up."

He said, "You have to learn to think differently."

I said, "It so happens that the way I think is the way I think, so how do I think differently?"

There was silence on the other end of the line. So I said, "A little louder, please! I can't hear what you're saying to me!"

His reply, "You will pray every day."

That was the best prescription I ever received from a doctor. It worked wonders, cost nothing and had only one side effect: peace of mind.

It was the only thing a person in a desperate situation could do. There are problems that only God can deal with, and He pulled me through. He planted some positive thoughts in my head. I knew things were better the day I looked at Dave and said, "I need to live to see Dan graduate from college and get married and then I'll think of another reason to go on." And it came to pass that Dan did get married to beautiful Stephanie and he did graduate from college, and I was there on both occasions.

At Dan's graduation I cried tears of joy because our daughter, Becky, and her wonderful husband, Japhet, had come all the way from England to Southern California for the event. I also cried because Becky was sick, morning-sick, and a beautiful grandson, Joshua Henry Crooker DeOliveira, was on the way.

Every day God has provided me with the desire and motivation to live. Was everything perfect from then on? Not exactly.

One morning Dave awakened me to say, "We've had a reversal." This was our code for any occurrence that could have negative consequences, financial or otherwise.

"What kind of reversal," I replied sleepily. He answered, "Our sewer has backed up into our house."

I was suddenly wide-awake and freaked-out. Having a sewer back up into one's house is no way to begin a day. I have a germ-phobia which stems from a microbiology class I took years ago while in pre-nursing.

The teacher warned us not to get too worked up about germs, citing the case of a student who became so germ-conscious he refused to sleep more than one night on a pillowcase because he was certain that germs had crawled out of his nose and mouth and onto the pillowcase during the night.

After a quick look at our floor-to-ceiling Mickey Mouse-decorated powder room, I was frantic. The sewer had backed up through the toilet and, after filling the powder room, flowed into the hallway. I said to Dave, "the minute you leave this house I'm going to shoot myself!"

He said, "I won't go to work then."

I answered, "You have to go. You have to take people on a tour today. But don't worry, I won't kill myself. I have to get this mess cleaned up and we need experts. Give me the phone book."

A healthy, happy young man – highly skilled in the matter of backed-up sewers – came to our house and went to work. He cut up the violated carpet, disinfected everything, set up machines to dry the wallboard and consoled me as I sat on a chair blithering about my germ-phobia.

"This mess isn't helping your phobia, is it?" The funny thing is that the experience put to rest some of my worst fears. I quickly saw how efficient the clean-up crew was. Several men cleared the blocked sewer line, even videotaping its insides. Others engaged in cleanup. And these men, dealing with the stuff on a daily basis, seemed to be living normal lives.

The day took a definite turn for the better when our wonderful friends rolled into our driveway. They had sold their home and purchased a motor home in which they were still traveling.

Juliette, bless her heart, cares for the sick. I mean really cares for the sick! She sends get-well cards by the dozens. She pays visits. And on this particular day she wanted to tell me about a new cure for Parkinson's: two tablespoons of flaxseed oil daily.

After trying it, I knew that I had better get well fast so I wouldn't have to continue with the 'cure."

When one has Parkinson's they had better get used to advice. It comes with the disease. One of my least favorite conversations was with a lady whose husband had unfortunately had a double misfortune – contracting the disease and, forgive me, having his wife as a caretaker.

She had become overly interested in the treatment of Parkinson's, deciding that his best hope for living a comfortable life lay in eating 75 percent of his food in a raw state and refusing any medications that seemed to work. The poor man died unable to move, yet she told me that her ministrations had "made such a difference in him."

When people implore me to try various "natural" remedies, I quietly remind myself that snake venom is "natural" and yet can be very deadly.

Also an interesting observation is that the folks who know just what to do would not have a clue if they were confronted with the problem themselves. One day I complained to my doctor that I was unable to drive. Without even one ounce of empathy, he looked at me and said, "Could happen to me anytime." The fact that he was still able to drive and also was about 14 years my senior seemed to totally escape him.

He was very fond of his "today is all you have" idea. It went like this. "All you have is today! If you are not happy today, shame on you—there is no tomorrow, might as well enjoy today!"

I never asked him what to do if I did not like today. It must have been that the mere fact that he was healthy, wealthy and held a respectable position in the community made him quite satisfied. I happened to know that very little things bugged him terribly; he was unable to tolerate a political view different than his own. After a few too many lectures about my attitude and today being all I had, etc., I wisely moved on, in an attempt to find a doctor who could make today a little more tolerable and maybe even allow me at least a crack at tomorrow.

We met some wonderful and interesting people during our experience with the sewer back-up. A supervisor named Clyde, who had been relegated to office work after suffering a back injury, came to the house after-hours. On his own time he consoled us and directed the workmen who continued with the cleanup far into the night. He was in his element and having the time of his life! We found this to be very refreshing indeed.

Restoring our home to normal was not a one-day job, of course. New carpet and sheetrock had to be installed. There was painting to do. It took two months to complete all the work.

Chapter Thirteen

BEFORE THE BATTLE

Doomsday was a wake-up call for me. I felt an immediate sense of urgency. I was 49 years old and with so many hopes and ambitions yet to fulfill.

The "Monster" Parkinson's is unpredictable and therefore defies any given strategy or time table. Some people afflicted with the condition do well for many years. Others go downhill rapidly.

Life and health are uncertain for everyone. For me, Parkinson's was a motivator. Friends and family were baffled by my drive. I needed to do everything NOW!

On Doomsday, my doctor handed me a packet of Eldepryl, then considered a "marvelous breakthrough" in the treatment of Parkinson's, with the potential to slow progression of the disease by 50 percent. Furthermore, it was not mind-altering.

The brochure that came with the starter pills showed a bucket of fluid with the fluid leaking out – a graphic way to show that people with Parkinson's lose the chemical dopamine. So, logic dictated that cutting the rate of dopamine loss would slow the progression of Parkinson's. Eldepryl would, the brochure said, cause the bucket to leak only about half as fast.

The image of the leaking bucket inspired me to take my Eldepryl with a faith bordering on obsession. I was supercharged and over-stimulated. For nearly two years, I worked day and night. Dave tried to sleep through my efforts and it was not easy for him, because he could hear me dragging furniture around the house, hanging and re-hanging pictures and doing anything and everything I could think of.

The only thing I never found time for was sleep.

After almost two years of frenetic living with this wonder drug, my neurologist told me the medicine was not all it was cracked up to be. It was in fact not much more than an amphetamine. He said a newer drug, Requip (Ropinirole HCl), might slow the progression of my disease to the point that in 20 years I might be no worse. Did I want to try it immediately or wait?

I replied, "I want it now, because I want to be the same in 20 years."

I asked if the drug was apt to make me mentally confused and he said I should try a sample to see if it did.

I said, "How will I know if I'm mentally confused if I'm mentally confused?"

He agreed that that was a good question, that those who act strangely might not realize they were acting strangely. The solution, he said, was to ask others to observe me.

So I tried the medicine and "others" found me so energetic they wondered if they should take the medicine, too.

I felt so good, in fact, that Dave and I decided on another mountain climb. It was the fall of 1998 and we were on a trip to England to visit Becky and Japhet. Early in November, we shocked the locals of Fort William, Scotland, by rolling into town, checking into a bed-and-breakfast and reconnoitering the landscape to determine if Ben Nevis, the highest mountain in the United Kingdom, would be a worthy climb for us.

Compared with Mt. Rainier, Ben Nevis is a mere foothill, being only 4,409 feet high. But size can be deceptive. Ben Nevis is known for pulling treacherous tricks on the unsuspecting. Nine days out of ten the summit is socked in with fog and clouds. Climbers have been known to step off the steep, east face because they can't distinguish the snow from the foggy thin air.

Although we were overjoyed at the thought of climbing the highest mountain in the U.K., almost everyone we talked to took a dim view of our proposed climb. For starters, we needed much warmer clothing. When we went to a local outdoor store to make our purchases, the clerks warned that what we planned was very dangerous indeed.

I went to a bakery to buy some pastries and casually mentioned that my husband and I intended to climb Ben Nevis the next day. The surprised clerk said, "Oh, you musn't go. There's fresh snow up there." I replied that I was glad to hear about the snow, because snow isn't as slippery as ice.

O.K., so the Scots didn't think climbing Ben Nevis was a stroll in the park. In fact, it could be downright treacherous. But it remained for the son of the Westhaven B&B owners to drive home the point.

"Ben Nevis," he said, "is only for experienced climbers."

I told him that we were. "My husband," I said, "is a forester and has climbed many major peaks." And I added that I myself had come close to reaching the summit of Mt. Rainier, which is more than three times as high as their little mountain. The young man was unmoved by my bravado. He suggested that if we were really going to attempt the climb, which he thought was foolhardy, we should stop by the local police station and inform the officers of our plans.

ALICE CROOKER

The next morning, we got up early and left a note for the B&B owners. The note informed them that we would be climbing Ben Nevis and would be back to West Haven by nightfall.

For a long time we were the only nuts on the mountain and the weather was wild. At times the wind blew so hard I thought I'd fall over. But whenever I looked around, I'd see sheep. And I vowed to climb far enough to at least get higher than the sheep! About halfway, we started to encounter snow and the dry snow blew around wildly in the wind.

We were maybe three-quarters of the way up the mountain when we saw two men coming up behind us. They overtook us quickly and we asked if they had climbed the mountain before. "Only about 30 times," one replied. When we asked if they were guides, they answered, "No, we're just two old fools. The weather's so wild today, we were just wondering if we should continue."

I said, "You can quit, but I have to keep going today because I have Parkinson's disease."

They wished us luck and decided to press on. We followed until Dave said it was time to stop for lunch. When we'd finished eating, Dave announced that we would go to the top of the next hill and then turn back.

I was so frustrated at the thought of once more failing to reach the summit of a mountain I truly wanted to climb that I angrily threw my sandwich down in the snow and said, "Oh great, here's another mountain for me to dream about."

Dave took off, with me behind him. He was climbing the last hill when I suddenly heard voices. Dave was talking with someone. He yelled down, "Come on, Alice, you're going to make it."

I struggled up the hill and there were the "two old fools," who looked more like angels to me. They had waited at the top for us.

They pointed me to the summit and said, "Go quickly and then get down fast. Here comes the whiteout." They added, "You should be very proud of yourself. Most of the people who live in that valley have never been up here. Good luck to you and good luck in life." Then they shook my hand. Wherever they are now, I wish they could know how much their words encouraged and blessed me.

By that time, the clouds were swirling in. We moved quickly to the summit marker, where I raised both hands high in triumph.

The descent was a joy! We ran into a party of three American young people, two of whom were determined to reach the summit. The third member, a young lady, was slowing them down. "Slow-motion" asked if we'd advise her to press on or to turn back. My quick answer was, "If you wish to live, turn back and we will help you down." She wisely followed the advice, because darkness was coming on and the walking appeared to be far more difficult for her than it had been for me.

We helped each other on the way down. Dave loaned the young lady his walking stick. Fortunately, she was staying at a hostel about half a mile before the trail ended. Since it was getting dark, we asked her to please call Westhaven and tell the proprietors that we were on our way down and there was no need to send a rescue team for us.

We found the perfect place for a "Victory Dinner," the restaurant in the fanciest hotel in town. We were barely seated when we spotted a man from England we had conversed with briefly during our descent. Dave said to the waitress, "That man over there climbed Ben Nevis today!"

The man was thunderstruck when the waitress went over and congratulated him on his feat. He asked, "How did you know what I did today?" And the waitress said, "Because those two people sitting over there told me." The man came over and introduced his wife. Success is so satisfying!

I made a screen display of the pictures we took on Ben Nevis and said, "If I end up in a nursing home, I will take the screen with me and if anyone tries to give me any guff I will point to the screen and say, 'Don't try to boss me around unless you've climbed that mountain."

Making ceramic dishes turned out to be a lifesaver of a hobby for me. My friend Florence got me started at a paint bar, and I found it very good therapy. For a time I'd forget all about Parkinson's disease.

Keeping busy solves many problems, of course, and I tried to be doubly busy as long as possible.

The year 2000 brought a marvelous grandson into our lives and gave me still another outlet. Becky and Japhet, parents of the newborn, had purchased a home in Hertfordshire, England and they told me they would be very happy to have me pay a visit and decorate the baby's nursery.

So I bought Peter Rabbit wallpaper at home, hauled it over on good old British Airways flight 048 from Seattle and then spent days working on my grandson's room.

During my visit I noticed that the kitchen of Becky and Japhet's house was small and dreary. I kept my opinion to myself until Becky came to visit us and said, "I don't like my kitchen!"

"Good," I said, with a sigh of relief. "Why don't you have Japhet tear everything out of it and I will come over and together we will remake it."

The fun began. When I arrived, they had figured everything out. Unless you have been to an Ikea in the UK you haven't really experienced Ikea. We took three cars. Japhet and Becky had one, I rented one and Japhet's dad, Jalvan, had one. Japhet led the way and I followed. Japhet is anything but a slow driver. But on this day he practically crept along – for him – and I doubt that I exceeded 90 miles an hour to keep up with him.

Even though we arrived at the store early, there was a line of people waiting outside. We loaded up three carts with kitchen fixtures and proceeded to the checkout counter. The beleaguered clerk had so much trouble trying to add up the merchandise in the carts that he had to call on another clerk to help him count and recount everything.

The poor clerk had not been blessed with a sense of humor. I kept trying to cheer him up by saying things like, "Oh, this is not a problem, just think of what it will be like when I decide to bring it all back for a refund." Each time I made a joke he would fix me with a look that was positively homicidal.

After what seemed a millennium we got the bill settled and tackled the hard part, which was trying to cram all of that stuff into three cars.

Attempting to describe the scene is difficult. It almost takes a video to do it justice. Visualize if you will a parking lot crammed with cars. People are trying to load their cars with merchandise. Everyone somehow manages to be right where someone else wants and needs to be. The English are very polite and will even excuse themselves if someone else should happen to step on their foot. But on this warm day, politeness has vanished and the sound of cursing can be heard. One man came out of the store, took one look at the mayhem and muttered, "What a nightmare. "

Had Japhet not been ingenious, it almost certainly would have been a nightmare. But he managed to load everything in three cars. Back home, we piled the boxes in the living room and I became very much acquainted with them, since I slept near them, stepped around them, opened them and assembled what was in them for what seemed like days.

We first tackled the ceramic-tile floor. The tiles were one of the few things we didn't buy from Ikea. The only thing I knew about laying tile was that you begin in the middle of the room and work out from there. Japhet and his father had located dead center and I began to lay tile. It is said that "fools go where angels fear to tread." My children are not fools, but I do believe angels are with them as they walk about on the uneven kitchen floor I provided for them.

Becky and I struggled to assemble the cabinets and quite literally worked day and night. When it finally came time for me to leave, it took my last ounce of strength to drive to Heathrow Airport, turn in the rental car and check in for the long flight home.

Then I heard words that my ears refused to believe. The woman at the counter said, "Take your bags and wait over there. We have no seats on the plane."

I had no energy left. I had used it all up in the kid's house. I said in a weak voice, "You will have to get help for me because I have Parkinson's disease and cannot move anything just now." The clerk called for help, had my luggage moved and even managed to get me on the flight. I sat next to a lady in great pain. She had broken her tailbone on the trip. We were good company for each other.

My period of superhuman strength was beginning to slip away. Once it began to go, it went fast. The most common advice to PD patients is: "Stay active. Keep going. Those who stay active do the best!"

I found out rather quickly that those who manage to stay the most active are probably in the early, mild stages of this strange disorder. In my case the motivation remained, but my strength was waning.

People ask what it's like to have Parkinson's. I say it's like walking underwater. The resistance to movement is very difficult to overcome. And it is extremely frustrating when it becomes difficult to maintain one's balance.

A sad fact I observed about being chronically ill is that as long as I put on a cheerful face and kept up, everybody loved and admired plucky Alice. But when the going got tough and I really needed help, it was easy to tell the true friends from the fair-weather ones.

Chapter Fourteen

LOSING THE BATTLE

CRASH! It was the sound of me falling headlong into the office bathroom.

Edward, my boss, immediately yelled, "Alice! Are you all right?"

Of course I wasn't all right. But I managed to scoot away from the wall my head had just slammed into and stagger out of the bathroom to come face-to-face with Edward, who was nearly as shaken as I was.

I said, "I really don't know how all right I am at this minute. But, while I sit on this chair and think about it, I'd be grateful if you could get some ice and put it on my head."

Upon hearing my request, poor Edward – who tends to be squeamish – summoned his daughter, Jizel, and told her to get the ice and hold it on my forehead. I asked both Edward and Jizel to please check my eyes to see if the pupils were the same size.

It was January 2002. Olympic Jewelers Ltd & Provident Loan Co., the Seattle firm that employed me, had closed its long-time downtown office and moved to new quarters atop a Banana Republic clothing store.

Edward, Jizel and I were the only survivors from our old crew. Before the mishap, I had been frantically trying to manually reconcile and close the books for the year 2001. It was not an easy task, because the company had held a giant going-out-of-business sale and I was inundated with paperwork.

My former helper in accounting had been caught embezzling big bucks and had very conveniently dropped dead of a massive heart attack the night before the cops planned to arrest her.

Accounting was a great profession for me. There were not very many dull times. I was trapped in the mist of a bank robbery in the Bank of America branch where I went daily to deposit cash receipts. Only after the police and FBI arrived was I allowed to leave the building. Oddly enough, this was the only premonition I have ever had in my life. As I stood in line waiting for a cashier, the idea strolled through my head that "You are in the banks a lot, Alice, what if a robber happens along?" According to eyewitnesses behind me, the robber was watching me intently. He was probably wondering which teller to go for.

Finally it was my turn to be waited on and I was chatting with the cashier, when an ashen-faced fellow cashier approached us and said, "I was just robbed!'"

"Oh no", I gasped. "Did he have a gun?"

"He told me to give him tens and twenties or he would shoot me and himself."

I am so grateful the robber did not say that to me, because with my stupid mouth, I would most likely have responded with "Please make certain you begin with yourself."

To add to the pressure at work that January, I was scheduled to fly to England later in the month to be on hand for the second birthday of our first-born grandson, Joshua, whom we were taking to Disneyland in Paris, France, to celebrate.

Another nagging problem was the seven-ton safe that the management of our "old" office insisted that we move "yesterday." I was in charge of finding a home for it.

And, finally, my Parkinson's disease – first diagnosed in 1996 –had begun to intrude on every aspect of my life.

At first I had attacked the disease with great vigor, determined to show everyone that it could be overcome. Now I was tired and spent precious time trying to keep from falling over. The reason I was seated in a chair awaiting an ice-pack on my forehead was that, unbalanced by Parkinson's, I had tripped on a step to the bathroom and plunged head-first into a wall.

My blue titanium-frame eyeglasses, which had landed on the tile floor, were in far better shape than I was. I made a note to extol the virtues of titanium frames to all my friends.

Despite a throbbing head, which felt no better after applying the ice than it had before, I knew I must return to work if I ever wanted to take my vacation.

I made it home, ate dinner and went to bed. In the middle of the night I got up and caught a glimpse of myself in the bathroom mirror. My eye was black and ugly. I looked terrible! Dave was awake enough for me to tell him the bad news. He answered, "Oh, I don't imagine you look that bad." But when he got up in the morning and took a look at me he realized I had not been exaggerating.

After two days of an unrelenting headache, my neck also began to hurt. I called Carewise, a medical service that decides when an emergency-room visit is called for. I described my plight and was told to have Dave wrap a towel around my neck and drive me immediately to the emergency room.

Off we went to Overlake Medical Center near our home. The attending physician, Dr. Eric Friedland, (Dave and I both love this personable and competent ER doctor and met him on other occasions) took one look at my eye and asked if I was on blood-thinners. I replied that I was not, since I managed to bleed profusely with no outside help.

Doctor Friedland asked why I had waited so long to seek assistance. I replied that I had been busy working and, since I had not vomited, lost consciousness or had a pain in the neck until now; I had seen no reason for alarm.

The doctor sent me off for x-rays of my neck. When the x-rays came back, he studied them and decided he wanted further pictures. I said, "I can't have a broken neck." He responded, "You crashed into a wall didn't you?"

When I got back to the emergency room, always calm and assured Dave had lost it. Between rants, he said, "Do you know what the doctor said? He said you need a CT scan of your neck before you can be cleared to go to London." In the future, he added, we should always listen to our friend Cherry who had warned immediately after my fall that I should go see a doctor.

While I was undergoing the CT scan, I made all sorts of promises to God, not the least of which was a lot of money for the church if he'd just let my neck be all right. As I was wheeled out into the hallway, the doctor approached, smiling, and said he'd studied all the pictures. The verdict: "I love your brain. I love your spine. Go to London."

My visit to England and France was a blast. Becky, Japhet, Joshua and I crossed the English Channel aboard a Hovercraft. Storms and choppy seas caused us all to become seasick, but Disneyland, Paris, was simply wonderful and Joshua turned two.

When I returned home my relationship with my neurologist began to sour. He didn't seem to relate to my balance problems, wondering aloud if I wasn't just being "klutzy" when I took all those tumbles. Things went rapidly downhill after I drove Dave to the airport one morning and then went to a doctor's appointment. I explained to him that I had taken an extra carbidopa/levodopa pill that morning because I didn't want to drive with "rigor mortis." Instead of giving me guidelines to deal with emergency situations he proceeded to scold me.

"You are never to take extra medicine," he said. "We will leave your medication the same."

The next year-and-a-half was a nightmare. I walked with extreme caution, leaning against walls to maintain my balance. The doctor continued to tell me I was doing just fine. If I complained, he would recommend a psychiatrist. I was not, in his words, "emotionally accepting my disease."

Kind people offering to assist me, gave me a funny look when I responded, "Thanks, but my doctor tells me I'm just fine."

Matters came to a head after I returned from yet another trip to England. Dave and I began preparations for a trip to Maui, so I felt a visit to the doctor was in order because I had, frankly, been quite limited in what I could do in England. I wanted to feel a lot better for our Maui adventure.

When I told the doctor I felt just awful, he cut me off and said I was the best Parkinson's patient he had and it was time I got used to some limitations. Once again he recommended a psychiatrist. I countered that I was crashing into walls. He responded, "Walk with a cane and get used to it."

Maui was worse than a disaster. The trip began with me nearly falling down in the security check at Seattle's SeaTac Airport. On Maui, I swam only one time – in the resort pool – and Dave had a difficult time getting me out. I spent the rest of the vacation time trying to remain upright.

I returned home very frustrated, finding it difficult to perform the simplest tasks. Some close friends were moving and I wanted to have a farewell dinner for them. I asked my friends Cherry and Juliette to come to our house and do all the work while I spent my time trying not to fall down. Both were horrified to see how my condition had deteriorated and insisted that I call the doctor. I had already asked him for a referral to the University of Washington Medical Center and had also made an appointment with Dr Russell Vandenbelt, a psychiatrist, at the doctor's request.

Dr Vandenbelt wondered why I was returning as he recalled that he had seen me previously and that I was just fine. When I told him my doctor felt I needed a psychiatrist to help me accept the limitations of my disease, the psychiatrist seemed skeptical.

Thanks to the prodding of Cherry and Juliette, I took a deep breath and decided to call my neurologist one more time. When I got him on the line, I informed him that I had previously been able to recover from operations, climb mountains and work all day and night. And now I was capable of doing virtually nothing. Hoping he would recommend an adjustment in my medicine, I asked him point blank what he would do if he were me.

The doctor said he saw no reason for me to come to his office. He ordered me to go to the hospital for a "psychiatric evaluation," and he repeated again that I had not "emotionally accepted my condition."

Then he asked, "Are you suicidal?"

I responded, "No!" He repeated the question. I repeated my answer and added, "I have told you it has entered my mind, but I do not do everything that I happen to think of." I protested that I did not need to go to the emergency room and furthermore I was at home alone with no car. He told me to call a cab. When I said I didn't want to do that, he made me promise to have my husband take me to the hospital as soon as he got home.

I have never been so mad in my entire life! But I decided to follow his advice to the letter to prove that it didn't make any sense. I called my insurance company and announced that my doctor had ordered me, against my wishes, to go to the hospital emergency room for a suicide analysis. I announced that I was not suicidal but would do what the doctor suggested.

When Dave arrived home from work, I greeted him by saying, "We have to go straight to the hospital to make sure I'm not suicidal."

Dave dropped me off at the emergency room and went to park the car while I lurched into the waiting room.

The startled receptionist said, "Let me get you a wheelchair."

I responded sarcastically, "Now why on earth would you do a thing like that? I have Parkinson's disease and I am here to see a psychiatrist. When the psychiatrist gets through with me, I will walk just fine."

After plopping me in a wheelchair, the receptionist gasped, "Your ankles are swollen."

I replied, "Don't worry; the psychiatrist can fix that, too."

The emergency room folks next wondered about my privacy rights, and I said, "I wish no privacy whatsoever. Call the news and broadcast this to the entire world. You can also put it on the web."

They took me to a horrible room. There was nothing on the walls and the bed looked miserable, with shackles for a patient's hands, feet and neck. "How lovely," I said.

"Someone will soon be with you," I was told.

Before "someone" arrived to see me, Dave walked in. I burst into tears. Suddenly, I quit thinking about myself. Dave looked so very tired. He had come home after a long day at work, had not had any dinner and it was getting late.

"This whole episode will make a great story for my book," I said. "So let's have some fun. I'll begin by telling you a joke."

Once upon a time a 15-year-old boy came home with a brand new Porsche. His parents freaked out and asked, "Where did that car come from?" The boy replied, "The lady up the street sold it to me for $15." The mother said, "Obviously she must be a child molester or an opportunist of some kind." She then implored her husband, John, to go to the neighbor's house to sort things out.

John walked up the street and discovered a pleasant lady planting petunias in her front yard. He asked, "Did you sell my son a Porsche for $15?" When she nodded in the affirmative, he said, "Why in the world did you do that?" "Because," she answered, "I just got a call from my husband and it turns out he is not on a business trip. He and his secretary are in Hawaii. They'll be there for the duration. He asked me to sell his Porsche and forward the proceeds, so I did!"

Shortly, a lady with black pointy-looking glasses appeared and I asked, "Are you the doctor?"

She answered, "No, I'm a social worker."

"Oh," I said, very expansively "What a lovely room this is. My husband and I are enjoying these beautiful surroundings."

She answered nervously, "Your doctor is concerned about your safety."

I said, "Oh, he is, is he? I would like to inform you that if a person were contemplating suicide, a depressing place like this could certainly drive her or him to go through with it."

Dave chimed in with, "Can't you at least hang a picture of Mickey Mouse on the wall?"

The poor social worker looked flustered. She didn't need this anymore than we did. I knew the laws of the State of Washington and was aware of my rights and I took full advantage of the situation, venting all my anger at my doctor on this poor woman.

I said again that it was a bleak place that resembled what I imagined Siberia must look like. Dave called it a "gulag."

I told the social worker my doctor probably wished I would kill myself since I was not an ideal patient. But I said I had absolutely no intention of doing anything of the kind.

I told the woman I had thought about doing a great many things in my life, but had not done them. That included strangling people and just then (I thought, but declined to say) the doctor was foremost in my mind.

She asked, "Do you want to hurt people?"

I said, "No, never."

She asked if I had ever tried to kill myself.

I said, "No, I like myself and suicide is against my religion."

The social worker looked at Dave to see if he would confirm what I said. Dave nodded his head. At this point, I got on my high horse and to the poor woman's shock rolled out my favorite Abe Lincoln quote "If I were a fool cut in half, I'd have better sense in either end than to try to end one war by beginning another."

I changed it to, "If I were a fool cut in half, I'd have better sense in either end than to be unable to think of killing myself."

The reason I had not done it was because of my great impulse control.

The frightened social worker ran from the room to call Dr. Vandenbelt to see if I should see him sooner. I told her to tell him that all was well, leave my appointment as scheduled. He went with my recommendation, not hers

I had just that day received a letter from a man dedicated to finding a cure for Parkinson's disease. He wanted funds for research. While I admire the man's efforts, his dismal picture of Parkinson's was a downer.

With that, I handed the letter to the social worker and said, "Here, look at this. Isn't it uplifting?"

This letter told about a man afflicted with Parkinson's who had lost his family, his hope and, of course, his interest in life. It ended with these words, "What would you do if you or someone you loved had this disease?"

Then I demanded to know why I couldn't see the neurologist. I said, "I want him to come down and stand in this pit and explain a few things to me."

She kept trying to persuade me to come over to their facility if at anytime I felt unsafe. I responded, "No way." I could not abide their dreary room and would have even preferred to wait out by the fish tanks in the lobby for the doctor.

In time, the emergency room doctor, not a psychiatrist, arrived. She was pregnant.

I tapped her on her wide belly and said, 'What do we have here?"

"A boy," she replied.

The doctor immediately grasped the situation when I said, "The only problem we have here is my Parkinson's disease. If it could have waited to afflict me until about 10 years after I'd died and been buried, everything would have been just fine."

The good doctor, who seemed to understand my quirky humor, said it was tragic I had come down with Parkinson's so early in life, I wanted to jump up and hug her.

They wrote on my chart, "Depression." I said, "Why am I depressed?

They said, "Because you have Parkinson's disease."

They discharged me and on the way home I told Dave, "Great! Now I can't even be president of the United States, because 'depression' is in my medical records." We both remembered when candidate George McGovern's running mate Thomas Eagleton had been forced off the ticket in 1972 due to a history of depression.

Soon afterward, I took Dave with me and went to see Dr. Russell Vandenbelt, psychiatrist and doctor extraordinaire. Dr. Vandenbelt, whom I had consulted once before, completely changed my opinion of psychiatrists. He is absolutely wonderful.

"What on earth happened the other night at the hospital?" he asked.

I answered that I had never been so angry in my life. All I did was ask my neurologist what he would do in my position – living with an ever-worsening case of Parkinson's disease – and he ordered me to go to the hospital to see if I were suicidal.

Dr. Vandenbelt said, "He thinks you're manic depressive, Alice."

Dave interjected, "I've never seen her depressed."

I told Dr. Vandenbelt that I had so many things I wanted to do with my life, including writing a book, that my neurologist thought I exhibited manic symptoms. I added, "All I need to do is have you talk me into my disease. And while you are at it, please get me to the point where I can get out of the car easily and walk around without falling down."

Dr. Vandenbelt said, "Let's get a second opinion on your Parkinson's." He referred me to Dr. Phil Ballard, chairperson of the Northwest Parkinson's Foundation. Dr. Ballard was now retired and doing only consulting work. People came from all over the world to see him.

Dr. Ballard had a very different take on my condition. I was not, he said, the best Parkinson's patient he had seen. In addition, I was severely under-medicated. What I needed was a doctor who would work with me.

Although my first neurologist's intentions were good, he failed to focus on my problem, which was Parkinson's disease and not suicide. He did a wonderful thing for me, however, when he referred me to Dr. Vandenbelt. As it turned out, he saved my life, not from suicide but from pancreatic cancer. Meeting Dr. Vandenbelt was one of the best things that ever happened to me in terms of my health. This doctor from day-one was on my side. He referred me to wonderful doctors and stuck up for me. He was right. Even when I began to doubt my own sanity, he did not.

A quick example: The following year I made several visits to the University of Washington Hospital's ER complaining of terrible abdominal and chest pain. They couldn't put their finger on the cause. During one visit they went to extreme efforts to save me from a suspected heart attack. I told them my heart was perfect, trying to save them trouble and expense. When they discovered I was indeed correct, they asked if I had a psychiatrist. They called Dr. Vandenbelt and even shared with me his response. He told them, "Sure she is anxious, something is wrong, keep looking. She is not crazy."

I changed neurologists and things improved. The reprieve was brief.

Christmas of 2003 should have been a delight. Before Christmas, Dave and I took Joshua to Disneyland and we had oodles of fun. Becky and Japhet were expecting again. This time they were told to expect a girl. They had decided to name her Mia.

But once again, Parkinson's reared its ugly head. I started "freezing," meaning I would be going along just fine and suddenly I would freeze up and be unable to walk. Dave rescued me when he found me stuck to a display in a Hallmark shop.

A quick visit to the new neurologist was the beginning of a real disaster. Disregarding the written instructions of Dr. Ballard, she adjusted my medication in the wrong direction. Dr. Ballard had suggested reducing the Requip and increasing carbidopa/levodopa, instead she increased both. I should have spoken up, but I didn't want to get on the wrong side of another doctor.

I was scheduled to leave in late February to go to England for the birth of Mia. Three weeks early, Joshua called and said, "Grandma, Mia isn't a girl. Mia is a boy."

Chapter Fifteen

LOOK'N GOOD

Since early childhood, my vanity had been thoroughly squelched. I had been studiously taught that I was ugly. My mother wasted not a penny on my clothing and simply gave me her cast off's, She provided me with clothing that was inappropriate and ill-fitting. While I slithered about looking and feeling like a total dork she lectured me about my attitude, inner beauty, etc., made certain I stood up straight and made it very clear to me how fortunate I was to have a mother who cared so deeply for me that she even spanked me. I would have much preferred that she show her great love for me in a far different manner.

At that time my mother was an average-size woman, I was tall and thin and my grade school teacher finally told Mom that I needed smaller clothes and preferably some dresses because they could hang from my shoulders instead of falling off my nonexistent hips. I should have told Mom that her clothes were too large for me, and to throw them somewhere else, but I lacked in two areas. I had no looks and obviously no guts.

My fourth grade teacher was not helpful either. I was but nine years old and I have never fully recovered from the shock of the observation she blurted out to me in front of the entire school as I was happily eating my lunch. The direct quote was

"When the looks were passed out in your family, you were passed by." OUCH!

I knew she spoke the truth because she liked me. She told everyone I was her best student and so smart I could be anything—even a doctor if I wished.

Worse than the teacher, was the Superintendent of Education.

She was a tiny, feisty, proper, bundle of energy—a very critical mass. She would strut into the classroom on her stilt high-heeled shoes, head held high and back ramrod straight. Her eyes darted about looking for the slightest deviation from total perfection and she always found it, in me.

She would begin to speak, usually about what a wonderful job of child rearing she had undergone and indicate there was no hope for us because we had not benefited from the wisdom and techniques of her parents. Somewhere in the midst of her tirade, she would catch sight of me and that was it. Drawing herself together, so as to look even more fearsome, she would hiss, "Alice Shumate, there you sit and your glasses are not resting on your nose properly, how can I possibly speak, or for that matter, even think with you in such a deplorable condition? You must and you will keep your glasses where they belong or I will glue them to your nose!"

She would then go back to her childhood dissertation and I was left amazed. How could this perfect lady, who was unable to tolerate anything out of order, ever have been a child? It seemed to me like she should have reared her parents instead of them her. She said another highly disturbing thing.

Speaking very precisely and emphatically she told us how proud she was of her father, because he was so dedicated to her that even when she was over 20 years old, she had spoken inappropriately in his presence and he had turned her right over his knee and walloped her. She doubted our dads would do that for us, and I hoped she was right.

It was impossible for me to keep my glasses up and listen to her so I went home and told Mom about the problem and she tried to help. She took me to an optometrist who took one quick look at my bridgeless nose, declared it "a very steep ski slope," and then said there was nothing he could do.

I once had a pair of pink glasses. Fortunately they had come to grief or this poor school administrator would have had even more to harangue about. In the '50s it was well known that red and pink did not go together. My hair was red and I don't know what possessed Mom to get me pink glasses.

I do know she was greatly relieved to discover I was only ugly and not stupid as well. She had finally sent me to school in the second grade at age seven and was very proud of my reading ability. However, at school I was unable to read the words on the blackboard. The teacher complained and when Mom asked me what was going on, I answered that I could not see. The eye doctor agreed and stated my eyes were an unusual combination. I was near sighted in one, far-sighted in the other and affected with astigmatism in both. The pink glasses gave the kids plenty to rag about and fortunately one day a little brat got mad at me and, yelled, "I will break your glasses!" Bam, she socked me and the pink glasses were history. They were replaced with blue.

When one is chosen, one is chosen. I was also chosen for crooked teeth. Obviously being ugly, having yucky clothes and a nose unsuitable for glasses was not nearly enough. I must have a mouth way too small for my teeth also.

Oh well, the old adage that one must be grateful for everything is true. At least I never wasted any time aspiring to be a model. I knew beauty wouldn't get me anywhere, so I worked on humor, charm, competency and reliability. I eventually discovered that in the adult world, most people don't really care what you look like, and if they like you, they like you. On the other hand, nice clothing and accessories can't hurt and may overcome a multitude of flaws. I was fortunate to marry Dave, who provided me money for clothes and jewelry.

I noticed I looked far better in a designer dress, coordinated shoes and carrying an expensive bag. In fact when I was chairing the boards, or telling a story to a large audience of children and adults, I found it very helpful to be immaculately and tastefully attired. If people are thunderstruck with your beautiful shoes, or diamonds, they will focus on them and not be able to devote so much time to you. For many years my looks were not an issue.

After I was diagnosed with Parkinson's everything changed. Suddenly, everywhere I went, people were awestruck by how wonderful I looked. I became amazed at how my looks magically improved. Things had gotten so bad that I was unable to even wear pantyhose. I would grab whatever would glide over my head, and shuffle about hoping no one would notice how awful I looked. My hair resembled that of a frightened porcupine, but wonder of wonders—lo, now I was so beautiful, so wonderful and such an inspiration. My friends would come and cheerfully say, "Alice you are looking so good today! How do you do it?" Then to someone beside us, "I don't know how she does it."

My weight had gone berserk and I was a pig. I could not do much of anything, so I did what I could do and that one thing was EAT!

The doctors gave up on me. They did not waste their breath by offering even so much as a hint that perhaps I could eat a little less. The doctors did not even wish to see me and spent inordinate amounts of time either telling me what a complicated case I was or how healthy I was. One doctor told me he wished all of his patients had my lab results. I felt like slapping him, but chose instead to move on.

The entire experience irritated and angered me. I feel for both sides. After all how can one relate to a person who still has her mind intact and is obviously on a downhill slide? I know now. Really, they are the same person. Whatever their interests were previously, they will remain the same. They will much prefer a stimulating discussion concerning just about anything to a patronizing, "My, don't you look marvelous!" I finally learned to just toss it back with a quick and light, "Well thanks, so do you!"

No one is to blame, but a serious disease such as PD will bring about changes. Everything will change, particularly relationships with friends and even family members. I refuse to go on a guilt trip over it. PD was not my idea or choice.

I let a friendship go over it. My friend liked to point out my faults, and treated me like a wayward child. I grew weary of the browbeating and let her know it. She acted as though I needed her expertise and advice every step of the way. She tried to tell me what to say to the doctors and even wanted a doctor to operate on me who had never even looked at me.

When she told me to just take a couple of Tylenol for a severe pain problem following a major surgery, I finally saw the light. She was a control freak and not a friend.

There is neither room nor inclination to fill this book with the surprises people have sprung on me when grasping for something meaningful to say. My least favorite query is, "Why are you different? You are not as much fun as you used to be!"

Chapter Sixteen

GOD'S WONDROUS WAYS

Today is October 6, 2004. In just seven days, Drs. Peter Nora and John Roberts of Virginia Mason Hospital in Seattle are scheduled to perform on me a procedure known as deep-brain stimulation.

This is how it came about:

The previous Christmas, a neurologist had adjusted my medication in the opposite direction from that recommended by Dr. Ballard. Shortly thereafter, I began experiencing a great deal of gastro-intestinal discomfort and our lives were consumed over the next few months with a search for the source of the problem. Dave and I went on a circuitous and baffling trip from doctor to doctor and ER to ER without finding any satisfactory answers and without anyone taking responsibility for my care – until I found Virginia Mason Hospital.

Let me make it clear that all of the doctors I have seen since the first signs of Parkinson's disease have wanted to help me. But like most of us humans, they get tired and discouraged and have limits to their knowledge and experience. Patients vary too. There are those who respond well to treatment and are a joy to work with. And there are others who, for various reasons, drive doctors to the brink of frustration.

Put yourself in their shoes. They have worked hard all day and finally managed to get some sleep. Then along comes one of those nuisances, like me, who seem to defy all efforts to diagnose, much less cure. And let's face it, not all doctors are created equal. Some are personable; others are not. Some are experienced and able to quickly assess a situation; others are not. But all have one thing in common: they are in the business of making patients feel better if at all possible. I turned out to be a double-barreled problem. Doctors not only couldn't make me feel better, they couldn't even settle on what was the matter with me other than I had Parkinson's. I was a challenge. All I knew was that I was sick, desperately sick.

The trouble began in England. Becky and Japhet's new baby, who they had been assured would be a girl, was now equally certain to be a boy. Or so the doctors said.

Becky and Japhet quickly decided that "Mia" would be named Jonah. Then they settled back to await the arrival of a Parkinson's afflicted grandmother who would step right in and care for Joshua, while they handled newborn Jonah.

Becky had recovered from the shock of the change in gender by the time I arrived in England, Feb. 25, 2004, bent on helping out. The flight had been hard on me, and I was pleased to accept wheelchair assistance to exit the plane. At the same time, I worried about Japhet's reaction when "helpful grandma" turned up in a wheelchair. Fortunately, my medicine kicked in quickly and I was on my feet by the time Japhet picked me up.

Becky was not feeling at all well, and here I came, noticeably impaired, hoping to make things easier for her. The way childbirth is handled in the United Kingdom differs considerably from what I was used to in the U.S. and I was petrified that Becky would give birth in the house. Joshua, had taken less than 8 hours to enter the world, and doctors assured her the second son would be considerably smaller.

On March 4, with still no sign of baby Jonah, I came down with a cold. At midnight, March 5, Becky's water broke and I insisted that she notify the hospital. She was told to come into the hospital immediately and I heaved a sigh of relief when she and Japhet left. They returned shortly, having been sent back home to wait until labor began.

Becky soon went into hard labor and I was anxious for her to start back to the hospital. She delayed, determined not to be sent home again. By the time she and Japhet left the house, her labor pains were so intense I was afraid she would give birth in the car.

The last thing I said was, "If the baby comes in the car, be sure to lie down so its neck doesn't break; meanwhile, I will pray."

They made it! Beautiful Jonah came into the world about 40 minutes after Becky reached the hospital. He weighed 7 lb. 1 oz. and Becky and Jonah came home that same day.

By the time Dave arrived five days later to see his new grandson, I was feeling much worse and Dave immediately began to worry. Besides worsening Parkinson's symptoms, I had terrible bloating and digestive difficulties. I thought getting home to my own bed would fix me up. So, with heavy hearts, Dave and I left our daughter, our son-in-law and our two beautiful grandchildren and headed home.

Our king-sized bed failed to cure what ailed me and we embarked on a never ending round of doctor's visits through the spring and summer that found nothing and fixed nothing. I was the "proverbial healthy horse." My friend Cherry decided it would be wise if I had my gall bladder removed. When I balked, she became downright snappish with me.

I finally said to her, "If you want it out, you had better come and take it out, because I can't just order it to be removed."

During this period of indecision, I developed a chill and both feet jerked involuntarily after I ate food or drank liquids. During an endoscopic exam my diastolic blood pressure dropped to 55. I was scheduled for a colonoscopy a few days later and because of my low blood pressure the doctor decided I should remain conscious during the procedure. Believe me this is something I would not recommend to anyone. I felt every twist and turn of the probe. Both of these procedures produced negative results.

Next was an abdominal CT scan with a tracer injected to produce contrast. The next weekend we went to a favorite restaurant for lunch with friends. I ate very little, but everyone was shocked to see my stomach visibly and painfully enlarge almost immediately. Even though it was the weekend, I called the gastroenterologist's office when I arrived home. I wanted some answers. An associate called me back. She had the results of the CT scan in front of her and she informed me that I had chronic pancreatitis. When I inquired how the condition came about the response was shocking: "Too much alcohol consumption."

I replied, "Thank you very much, I don't even drink."

Now I had two terrible conditions to worry about – Parkinson's disease and chronic pancreatitis. When I searched the web for information on how to deal with pancreatitis, it wasn't much comfort to discover that the remedy is to stop drinking alcohol. How could I stop drinking if I had never started? More troubling for Dave and me were the questions crowding our minds about what this condition meant and what if any treatments were available.

It was a long weekend of worry and, alas, when we visited my gastroenterologist on Monday he was no help. We asked about the results of the CT scan and the diagnosis of chronic pancreatitis. He was dismissive and said something to the effect that we, meaning the medical profession, don't know much about the pancreas.

My condition did not improve. There were still more tests, and I continued to have episodes of a lot more chilling and jerking and abdominal bloating. Dave remembered his vow to do what Cherry said and started in on the gastroenterologist by quizzing him concerning my gall bladder.

"Oh, her gall bladder is just fine," enthused the doctor.

"What is the definitive test and have you done it?" Dave was becoming persistent. Lo, the definitive test was an HIDA scan, a nuclear test that provides a visual display of gall bladder function. This test had not been done so the gastroenterologist ordered one for me before he left on vacation. I failed the HIDA scan miserably, my gallbladder showing no function whatsoever. I was told by the technicians to find a surgeon and have my gall bladder removed immediately. I readily agreed and quickly contacted Dr. Eiji Minami – a personal acquaintance and reputedly one of the best surgeons in the area.

We thought that at last we had found an answer to the problems I was experiencing. But after the operation, Doctor Minami said he didn't think the operation would cure my problem. He was right!

The gastroenterologist I was seeing just about defies description. He was the most charming, pleasant, personable air-head I have ever had the pleasure of meeting. He must have lied and cheated his entire way through medical school.

My problems persisted and he did not know what to do and he did not seem to have the wherewithal to find out. In spite of the fact that I had lost about 24 pounds, had no luck eating, or sleeping, he told Dave on the phone one night that he had no more ideas. Thank heavens we had at least one idea left; find a different doctor. A doctor who could sort through my baffling symptoms and who was willing to take responsibility for my welfare was what we longed for.

This book would never end if I recounted all my visits to doctors and emergency rooms and all the calls placed to the fire department on my behalf in the next three-and-a-half months. All we really learned is that I am extremely sensitive to drugs.

My neurologists determined that none of my problems had anything to do with Parkinson's. On the other hand, my doctors assured me that my problems had everything to do with Parkinson's, adding that my pancreas could act up at any time and cause me excruciating pain.

I was petrified that I might have cancer, since the symptoms of pancreatic cancer are similar to those of pancreatitis. And drinking does not bring on pancreatic cancer.

In desperation, I called the one doctor I had come to trust throughout this ordeal – psychiatrist Dr. Russell Vandenbelt. I asked if he could suggest a doctor who specialized in gastro-intestinal disorders, in hopes of discovering whether a pancreatic disease was at the root of my problems. Dr. Vandenbelt directed me to Dr Geoffrey Jiranek at Seattle's Virginia Mason Hospital. This was the doctor we had been looking for.

Dr. Jiranek has a heavy schedule and at that time was away on vacation so the earliest appointment we could get was over a month away. While waiting to see Dr. Jiranek, I made many visits to the University of Washington Hospital's emergency room. I was treated wonderfully. On one occasion a team of doctors worked hard to stave off what appeared to be a possible heart attack. It wasn't, but they continued to try to figure out what was causing my diverse symptoms. Our life was a nightmare. We could never sleep through the night and went from primary care doctor to ER to neurologist never finding out what to do and always being told we should be "somewhere else." Invariably, a new pill was prescribed and I would have another drug reaction. I would either react to the new drug or the withdrawal of a previous one. We used to laugh and say it would be fun to gather every doctor in the world together and say "Fix Alice." We thought the fight that would ensue when the opinions collided would be hilarious.

When I finally saw Dr. Jiranek, I was having an adverse drug reaction. When he heard my slurred speech, he immediately made an appointment for me to see a speech therapist. He was concerned about the cyst on my pancreas, stating that it was of unknown origin and we needed to find out what was going on. He scheduled me for a fine-needle aspiration; a procedure that inserts a needle through the stomach wall into the pancreas to remove fluid from the cyst. During the procedure it was discovered that I had not one but two cysts on my pancreas. There was no sign of pancreatitis. The cysts were drained and my situation improved. Best of all, he said there was no connection between the condition of my pancreas and alcohol drinking. It was so encouraging to have a doctor with intelligence, charm and a desire for facts and action.

The speech therapist that Dr Jiranek referred me to is Roberta Kelly in the neurology department. This charming, efficient lady should have killed me many times over, but guess what? I am still alive and writing this book. I was so sick, I missed the first appointment. No problem, they would make another one. I missed that one also. During one of my discussions with the office staff over a missed appointment, it was suggested that I might want to see Dr. John Roberts, who was, they said, "a wonderful, talented and caring neurologist." Dr. Roberts turned out to be all of the above, giving me my first ray of hope since the day I was diagnosed with Parkinson's.

During my first appointment, Dr. Roberts brought up the possibility of my undergoing deep-brain-stimulation to relieve the symptoms of Parkinson's. Dave and I had come to the appointment hoping I could be a candidate for DBS. I jumped at the chance. Dr. Roberts cautioned that there were several steps to go through to determine my eligibility, but that he thought I was an excellent candidate and that I had a realistic chance of responding well – meaning my off time could be reduced drastically. In the meantime he adjusted my medication so I could get a good night's sleep again. He significantly reduced the amount of Requip and increased carbidopa/levodopa in line with Dr. Ballard's recommendations a year earlier.

Dave and I were scheduled to take a cruise to Alaska aboard *The Norwegian Star*. In spite of my condition, but buoyed by the prospect of the brain operation, we decided to go for it. I am certainly glad we did. On the second day, we encountered gale force winds and heavy seas. Many of the passengers became seasick, but Dave and I seemed to thrive on rough water. Our only problem was my poor balance. One evening I crawled to the dining room door and then had Dave call for a wheelchair, since I didn't want to crawl to our table.

The dining room staff treated us royally that night, because many of the passengers didn't show up due to seasickness.

Dave spent much of his time caring for me on the cruise, and it was obvious that going back to work would be a vacation for him. Furthermore, it didn't appear there would be a peaceful retirement in his future unless the brain operation was successful. Nothing was easy for us on the cruise. Every time we left the boat we wondered if we would be able to return.

One evening Dave accidentally munched my evening's dose of Parkinson's medicine along with some popcorn. I panicked, called sick bay and said, "My husband might die." Fortunately, I think Dave managed to spit most of the medicine out because he developed neither the double-vision nor the "weird sensations" we were told might occur.

The prospect of the upcoming surgery gave us both hope. When fellow passengers would look at me sympathetically I would just say "I'm going to have a brain job and after that I'll be all right." That would lighten the moment immediately and you could visibly see them relax. It was great to have something positive to say about a dismal situation.

How do I feel today, one week before my surgery? I am thankful to my Mother who, despite our differences, continues to be an inspiration to me. God brought her through an extremely destructive brain surgery. Anything that I might face would be "duck soup" compared with what she underwent.

As I contemplate the deep-brain-stimulation surgery that lies ahead, I calm my fears by remembering God's promise: "I will never leave you or forsake you."

God knows what is best for me and I want His will to be done concerning the outcome of this surgery and in all other aspects of my life. I can now honestly say, "Not my will, but God's be done."

Chapter Seventeen

THANK GOD!

Hello again!

I know what you're thinking. You thought you'd finished the book and could say, "Good-riddance to that woman who's drowning in self-pity." You also may have vowed not to read any more non-fiction for awhile. Fiction is much more pleasant.

But here I am again. Today is October 29, 2004, and you will never believe how happy I am as I flit around the house, triumphantly testing my ability to stand on one foot at a time, amazing my family and friends.

With every breath, I praise God. I mail thank-you notes to my wonderful friends and family for all the beautiful flowers, prayers and kind wishes they sent my way.

I am bursting to tell you the rest of the story.

I first heard about the deep-brain-stimulation operation for Parkinson's disease on a television special several years ago. It seemed unreal that in the fall of 2004 I was hoping and praying that I would qualify as a candidate. After extensive neuro-psychiatric testing to determine if I was psychologically up to the procedure and a conference with the neurosurgeon to see if my brain was anatomically suitable (it is necessary to visualize the subthalmus clearly for the procedure), I was given the go-ahead for the surgery. Oh joy!

On Monday, Oct. 11, Dave and I went to Lindeman Pavilion at Seattle's Virginia Mason Hospital to sign consent papers for the operation, which would be performed two days later by Drs. Peter Nora and John Roberts.

Our calm was briefly shattered when we heard a receptionist say on the phone that Dr. Nora had undergone an emergency appendectomy the previous Friday. Would the operation have to be re-scheduled? Couldn't anything go right for us? This time things went our way. Although Dr. Nora's surgeries were being re-scheduled, one wasn't. Mine!

I signed the consent forms and relaxed further when Dr. Nora appeared, standing upright on both feet. He assured us that despite his recent surgery he would see me in two days. I looked at him and said, "You poor thing! But maybe this is a good omen. The doctor who delivered our second child was recovering from a hernia operation."

It would be nice to say that I was brave and calm prior to the surgery. But that would be a lie. I have never been so petrified in my life. All I could think of was brain hemorrhage, death or spending the rest of my life totally incapacitated. I was not encouraged when a nurse informed me that my blood was a bit thin, adding, "But we'll deal with it."

Worries about my upcoming surgery caused Dave to have panic attacks at work, but he didn't want to share his fears with me. I called our son Dan and asked him to come to our home and help Dave get me out of the house early on the morning of the surgery. I was instructed to be totally off my Parkinson's medication the morning of the surgery and at this stage of the disease, I was totally immobile in the mornings and would be a handful. (Dave's first order of business in the morning was to get me upright, then put medicine in my mouth and after about one-half to one hour I could walk around for a while). I wanted to ask Dan's wife Stephanie to come too, but since she was in nurses' training I didn't want her to miss any classes. She decided to come with Dan without being asked, and I was so happy to see her. Daughter Becky called from England and said the South England and British Union Conferences of the Seventh-day Adventist Church had just offered special prayers for me.

Suddenly I felt as if the whole world was on my side, although you'd never have known it to hear me. All I could say on the way to the hospital was "murder, murder, murder!" Dave said, "Can't you say something more positive?" I answered, "I'm so miserable I can't." My state without medication was truly frightful. I had been instructed to take no medicine after midnight, although Dr. Roberts said I could sneak one pill at 5 a.m. I decided I had one crack at this surgery and would hold off on all medicines. I was totally "stove up" (as in aching, cramped joints) before the surgery. My left hand was curled so tight it hurt. I doubt that I could have let loose of anything I was holding. I used to warn Dave before we went to sleep at night to be careful that my hand didn't get curled around his neck.

When we arrived at the hospital at 5:30 a.m., our wonderful pastor Phil Lizzi and his wife Judy were there to pray with me. I will be forever grateful to these dear folks as this meant they had to arise very early and travel to the hospital to be with me.

The surgery prep began. The anesthesiologist looked at me as if I had gone berserk when I opened my mouth and said, "Dr. Peter Nora had his appendix out on Friday." The distinguished anesthesiologist gave me a condescending look and said in a stern voice, "I have heard of no such thing!" He obviously thought I was hallucinating. I repeated what I'd said and vowed it was the truth.

The moment Dr. Nora arrived, the anesthesiologist said, "This lady insists you had your appendix removed last Friday! Is she correct?"

Dr. Nora replied, "Yes, she's right. I tried to keep it very quiet. That's why you didn't know."

There were so many doctors, interns and nurses working on me that I decided to relax by telling them a joke. I said, "Have you heard the one about the doctor who was testing three little old ladies for dementia? He asked the first, 'What's 3x3?' She snappily replied, '297!' Disappointed, the doctor put the same question to the second patient. She quickly responded, 'Friday!' He then asked the third patient, who correctly answered, '9.' Delighted, the doctor asked how she arrived at the answer. 'Simple,' she replied, 'I just subtracted Friday from 297.'"

When it came time for me to be taken into the surgery, Dr. Nora joined in hoisting me off the gurney. Alarmed, I said, "You stop right now! If you don't quit lifting me, you'll pull your stitches out." It must have been the smartest thing I'd ever said, because every doctor and nurse immediately agreed with me.

Dr. Nora backed off and said, "O.K. From now on there will be no further word about my surgery. The only thing we will concern ourselves with is this surgery and this patient."

Deep-brain stimulation is exactly what the name implies. The surgeons would be going deep into my brain to perform a procedure designed to make my faulty circuits function more reliably.

The operation began with a metal halo being positioned around my head and screwed into my skull. Then my head was shaved. Dr. Nora had said the halo placement would be the most painful part of the surgery and he looked worried when he saw the halo was crooked. It had to be unscrewed, repositioned and screwed into my skull a second time. Not the best way to start.

A dime-size hole was drilled in the top of my head, on the right side. I sensed the vibration and heard the noise, but felt no pain. When the drilling ended, Dr. Nora said, "You need to get her blood pressure down. We can't enter her brain with the pressure (185/110) this high."

They tried to reduce my blood pressure, but it remained high. Dr. Nora sighed and said, "She's resisting any effort to lower it." I did so want him to continue, so I began to pray, "Dear God, please save me and bring my blood pressure down." And down went my blood pressure.

Dr. Nora then entered the first hole drilled in my head and started inserting a thin cluster of wires into my brain. After a time I heard Dr. Roberts say, "I think we are in the subthalmus now." I heard static, and soon – quite miraculously—my tightly clenched left hand relaxed. Dr. Roberts then began questioning me. He asked me to say the days of the week and I started with "Today is Wednesday, Oct, 13, 2004." Then I thought, "Alice, he said to say the days of the week." So I said, "Sunday, Monday, Tuesday, Wednesday, Thursday, Friday and Saturday. He asked me how many clocks I saw on the wall. I replied that I saw two; one white and one black. He said that was correct and that if I had seen more it wouldn't have been good.

Dr. Nora then started drilling a second dime-size hole, this time on the left side of the top of my skull. His only comment was, "My, you have a thick skull."

My response was, "Thank you for that observation. Now, at last, I'll be able to explain to my friends and family why I am so stubborn and they can't get anything in my head."

Every so often I'd feel liquid running in my brain, and I'd ask Dr. Nora if it was blood or water. It was comforting to hear him say, "It's only water from my drill."

After the second hole was drilled and another cluster of wires inserted in the subthalmus, the first part of my surgery was complete. Dr. Nora heaved a gentle sigh of relief and said, "It's over and it's only 11:30."

That was the most frightening observation to me, because I looked at the clock and thought, then Alice, why do you see 12:00?

Rather than suffer endlessly I spoke up and said, "I am worried about my cognition. You said it is 11:30. Why when I look at it does it appear to be 12:00?"

The swift and welcome answer was, "Your cognition is fine, that is not a clock and the hands are in the 12:00 position."

One week later, the wires would be permanently connected to battery-operated neurostimulators that would be implanted in my chest.

An attendant pushed my bed from the surgery into a public elevator, which would take us up to the 17th floor. There, I would reside in a private room known as the penthouse of Virginia Mason Hospital. When we entered the elevator, people nearby gaped at me in horror.

I must have quite a sight with a shaved head and bandages on the top of my skull. I decided to enjoy my moment in the spotlight by saying, "Hello, folks! I just had a brain job and I'll have you know you are in the most wonderful hospital in the entire world." Several people decided to humor me by saying, "Oh, yes, we can see that!" and "Good luck to you!"

With just the wires implanted there was reported to be a "honeymoon" effect and I experienced this. Somehow, the initial implant of the leads gives some of the same beneficial effects provided by the neurostimulators. This can last from several hours to a day or more. Dave was very happily surprised when he came to the hospital to collect me and I was not in my room. He saw written on my blackboard, "This is a wonderful place!" and was further shocked to see me walking just as I had walked about ten years previously.

After a night of excellent care, I returned home. One week to the day, I returned to Virginia Mason for the neurostimulator implants. I was out cold for this and glad to be oblivious to what was going on. I regained consciousness very slowly. Upon awakening I found a towel draped over my head and a heat lamp shining on me.

With David hovering over me as I lay on a gurney, we both became aware that it was almost 5 p.m. – and I had a 5 p.m. appointment with Dr. Roberts on that very day. What to do?

While we stood there fretting, up walked Dr. Roberts. He seemed amazed that I hadn't realized he would see me in the hospital at 5 p.m. I wasn't supposed to come to him in my condition.

The moment we'd all been waiting for occurred when Dr. Roberts leaned over and turned on my neurostimulators. First he turned on the right side and made a few adjustments on his monitor. My left hand relaxed and quit curling and hurting. He then turned on the left side. It was a low voltage to begin with. I was quite weak and tired out and did not get up and run around like they do on the TV shows, but that operation was nothing short of a miracle. It was a quietly dramatic moment and never since that time has Dave had to arise at night and drag me to the bathroom. I am able to walk unassisted.

I went back to Dr Roberts several times and he turned up the voltage and lowered my medicines. My medicine has been drastically reduced! Requip has been eliminated and carbidopa/levodopa cut in half. This last November, 2005, Dave and I traveled to England on a business trip. The "business," was to purchase a darling second home in the backyard of our precious grandchildren. While we were there, Becky and I walked 4 miles roundtrip from her home to the Marlowe's Shopping Center. I often feel like pinching myself to make certain this is all real. Only in my dreams did I think I would be able to do that again.

Unfortunately, this surgery is not a permanent cure. The neurostimulaters will need new batteries in about three years. No problem. Deep brain stimulation should remain effective for about 10 years, perhaps more. Maybe there will be another medical miracle on the horizon by then. (Update January, 2006: a long term study has established good long-term effects for DBS and this good news can be found on the APDA website).

Sadly, while the surgery performed on me is the greatest breakthrough in the treatment of Parkinson's in the past 30 years, it doesn't work for everyone. Furthermore, many doctors seem inexplicably unaware of the procedure, so it is grossly under-utilized.

Looking back on my ordeal, I certainly am not grateful that I contracted Parkinson's disease. It did not make me a better person, nor was it a blessing for my family. I would like to campaign against Parkinson's disease until it is banished from the planet. Knowing that won't happen immediately, I would like to tell the friends and relatives of those who have Parkinson's disease to face the facts head-on. Knock off the "It-could-be-worse garbage!" We don't want to hear it.

A wonderful physical therapist told me that of all the neurological diseases with which she might be afflicted she would choose Parkinson's.

I responded, "Yes, it's such a marvelous disease that you could be dead for 5 years before anyone noticed you'd passed on."

She looked at me and, realizing the awful truth of my comeback, said simply, "You are so bad, Alice!"

I think the real reason doctors spend so much time telling patients how much worse it could be is because they are petrified when faced with a case of Parkinson's. Many haven't a clue as to how best to deal with its victims' roller-coaster emotions or how to provide a satisfactory treatment.

The wonderful thing about Dr. John Roberts, who is still my doctor, is that he is a busy man. His job is to get people better. He doesn't waste a moment saying, "It could be worse. Wear flat shoes. Adjust emotionally to your condition."

Let's wrap it up this way. If you have Parkinson's disease, you are in for it. You need help and you need it fast. Put first things first. Start with God. God is good. God is love. Ask God to help. He never fails. Then do not rest until you have found the best neurologist possible.

I am so glad God led me to Seattle's Virginia Mason Hospital and graciously provided Drs. Roberts and Nora to assist me. God can help you, too. May He bless you and keep you.

I'm an accountant, so I like things to balance out. To me, the bottom line is this:

PARKINSON'S DISEASE IS NOT GOOD
BUT GOD TRULY IS!

Chapter Eighteen

ODDS & ENDS

And you thought it was all over, that after scoring a technical knockout over Parkinson's, nothing bad would ever happen to me again.

Well, let's face it. I am a chronically ill person, never looking, but always finding a new ailment to adopt as my own.

A few months after the successful deep-brain procedure enabled me to take back my life from Parkinson's disease, I was having trouble again with my pancreas. Prior to the deep-brain procedure, I had been treated for not one but two cysts on my pancreas.

It came time to take another look at my pancreas and Dr. Jiranek performed another fine-needle aspiration. He called a few days later to say he was not pleased with the results and wanted me to see a surgeon. We scheduled an appointment for a week or so later.

After a few days of dreadful suspense, Dave decided to act. He said, "Let's go on a trip. We can drive around the North Cascades Highway." I immediately agreed. The weather was superb and the scenery in Washington State was, as always, unbeatable.

We stopped in the Bonanza-like town of Winthrop in Eastern Washington and ate scrumptious ice cream, then spent the night in a beautifully timbered lodge in the little town of

Soap Lake. The theme of our room was Odds & Ends, a truly amazing coincidence since I had already decided to title my final chapter Odds & Ends before Dave suggested the trip.

For breakfast, we went to a favorite little haunt in Dry Falls, and proceeded to laugh ourselves silly over absolutely nothing. When we arrived back home, we prepared for the now familiar trip to the Virginia Mason Hospital.

We were fortunate to meet the world renowned Dr. L. William Traverso, who educated us on the functioning of my pancreas. It was so heartening to have a doctor who actually knew something about the pancreas. The short version was that I had a 50/50 chance of having cancer. If I had cancer, it was probably contained, but there would be follow-up treatments and we were aware that the survival rate for pancreatic cancer is not high. He recommended removal of 40 percent of my pancreas and probably my spleen in the process.

I quickly agreed and said, "You can quit now and go on to something else." I knew he was taking a group of Italian doctors around the hospital and there was really no reason for him to spend more time with me. Dave wanted to know more, however, and foremost among his concerns was that I would be a diabetic following the surgery. Not to worry. Dr. Traverso said there would be plenty of pancreas left to do the job.

And so it came down to a coin flip. I had even odds of the cysts being cancerous or benign. If it was cancer, and it was contained, I had a 55 percent chance of surviving five years, because Dr. Traverso and Virginia Mason are the best on the planet. My odds would have been less at most other hospitals. If there was no cancer present, I would be all right.

Parkinson's disease is rough and tough, but it certainly prepares one for the prospect of dying. All I could say was, "I would rather go quickly with pancreatic cancer than return to the state I was in before the deep-brain-stimulation therapy operation."

Then I added, "God knows what lies ahead. I do not," which is exactly how I felt on June 1, 2005, when Dr. Traverso operated on me.

After two days of nail-biting (mostly by Dave because I was too miserable to worry much) the lab results came back: precancerous, but no cancer at this time. Dr. Traverso emphasized, however, that it had been a close call.

My thoughts on the matter: God must have something He wants me to do here on Earth. I want to find out what it is and do it. While I'm looking, I think it might be fun to find another hobby, something totally unrelated to doctors, emergency rooms and surgeries.

Oh yes, my first draft of this chapter contained a mock letter to the unnamed gastroenterologist who once hinted my pains were probably all in my head and, besides, why was I going on about the pancreas "which nobody knows much about anyway."

Of course the letter was never sent, because there's already too much meanness in the world. But I was happy when my editor called and said, "Would you mind not using that letter in your book?" After confessing to him that writing the unmailed letter had been therapy enough, I agreed.

He laughed and hit the delete key.

Another real miracle here was that a CEA level had been requested for the original pancreatic cyst biopsy, but not supplied. The CEA level on the second was 2091—normal is just under 20. It was probably out of sight on the first test also and might have disqualified me for the Deep Brain Stimulation operation. Without that I would have not made it through the distal pancreatectomy and splenectomy!

Wayne Dyer in his book "The Power of Intention" writes and talks about how the way we look at something will change it, and he is so right. When I replaced thoughts of anger at the doctors for not sorting everything out sooner, with thoughts of what might have been if they had, I saw a real blessing.

THANK YOU

Thank you for purchasing and reading this book. You have helped the PD Community because the proceeds from this book are being donated to the Virginia Mason Hospital Foundation and earmarked for the Neurology Department. You now know a lot about how I think and live. I have much to be thankful for and I hope this book has been of encouragement to you.

Having PD has opened my eyes to the incredible kindness of most people and also to the need for self-improvement. It has been a real revelation to me to find out just who my real friends are and I am happy to report that contrary to conventional wisdom, PD will not cause the end of a well- founded and firmly grounded friendship,

People have surprised me with their outpouring of love and goodwill. I will never forget the day in the Virginia Mason Hospital when a young lab assistant, whom I had misjudged because of his appearance, nearly started to cry as I related to him my difficulties. He said, "Lady, I am going to pray for you."

A few, very few, people have not been nice, but they simply missed an opportunity and a blessing, so why waste time worrying about them? I have more, far more, to be thankful for than most folks. Everyday that I wake up is a bonus, a day granted to me by God and my prayer each day is that I can help someone. This prayer is always quickly answered. I am grateful to God He has never, not for a second, turned His back on me or let me down. What God has done for me, He will do for you or anyone else who asks for His help.

Whatever difficulty you are experiencing, please don't try to deal with it alone. The wonderful truth about God is that you don't even have to explain to Him your problem or your needs. He already knows. All He needs to hear from you and from me are the words, "Dear Lord, please take me in your arms and help me."

You say, "I have no faith in God." God knows that and He will give you faith. God knows exactly when and how best to help you.

Also, thanks to God, I am assured that this life is not the end. I look forward to a heaven in which all things are new.

My final thoughts on trouble are that the only one who can truly help you is God. So find him now. It will not be difficult because He is looking and longing for you.

GOD IS SO GOOD!!

Please visit me at my website: **www.freewebs.com/ acrooker/** I would love to hear your story!

Printed in the United States
55631LVS00002B/190-240